Gallstones:

Ridding Stones Naturally

In 24 Hours!

By Dr George J Georgiou, Ph.D.,D.Sc (AM),N.D.

Dedication:

First, I would like to give any thanks and a bow to the thousands of patients who have helped me understand the complexities of chronic diseases - for placing your trust in me, and allowing experimentation when things were not so clear.

All these patients over the years have been my "laboratory" for developing many treatment protocols through trial and error, backed by research.

I would also like to thank all the researcher scientists, lecturers and teachers who dedicate their life to helping others, and all the courageous health professionals who go against the grain of the establishment, while thinking outside the box. Specifically, I would like to mention a colleague and friend who departed us last year, Andreas Moritz who wrote one of the first books on the Gallbladder Flush – you have left a legacy behind you, dear Andreas!

A loving hug of gratitude to my wife and 4 children for their support and understanding during my professional endeavours throughout these years – they are all blessed.

Finally, I deeply embrace the Divine faith that I have been blessed with, that has helped me believe in the innate healing abilities of the body, through the power of Natural healing, without chemical intervention.
A profound blessing to you all and may your healing journey be fruitful and fulfilling!

Published by
Da Vinci Health Ltd
Panayia Aimatousa 300
Larnaca, Aradippou 7101
Cyprus

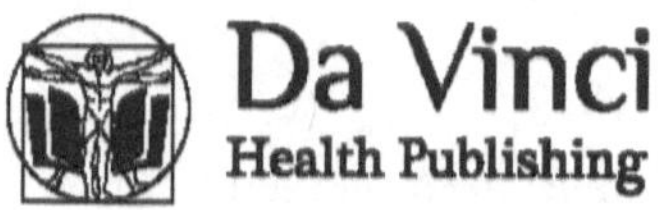

ISBN: 978-9925-569-04-5

TABLE OF CONTENTS:

CHAPTER I:

GALLSTONES

There is no scientist that will dispute the fact that **WE ARE ALL TOXIC!** We live on a planet where we are exposed to over 100,000 toxins, with an additional 1,000 added *each year*.

It is the liver that helps to detoxify all these toxins or xenobiotics as they are often called. If you didn't have a liver, you would be dead in less than a few days – mainly because of toxic overload.

The liver is the gateway to the body and in this chemical-age its detoxification systems are easily overloaded. Thousands of chemicals are added to food and over 700 have been identified in drinking water. Plants are sprayed with toxic chemicals, animals are injected with potent hormones and antibiotics and a significant amount of our food is genetically engineered, processed, refined, frozen and cooked.

All this can lead to destruction of delicate vitamins and minerals, which are needed for the detoxification pathways in the liver. The liver must try to cope with every toxic chemical in our environment, as well as damaged fats that are present in processed and fried foods.

Therefore, it is crucially important to cleanse your liver regularly, much like you clean your house, car and external self. Cleansing once per year is a good thing. When the liver gets overloaded it cannot metabolize fats and cholesterol so easily, and this is when your cholesterol starts creeping up. But also, the liver itself becomes "fatty." Fatty livers are usually found in about 50% of people over the age of 50; this is often seen by radiologists examining people routinely. Any imbalances in the liver will have a direct effect on the gallbladder, as it is the liver that produces the bile and gallstones.

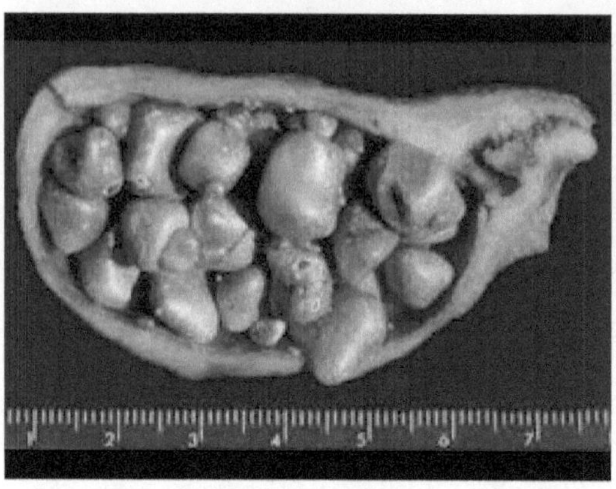

Before we look at the fascinating structure and function of the liver, I would like to look at the gallbladder and how this organ can be easily cleaned with amazing health benefits.

The Gallbladder and Disease
The gallbladder is a pear-shaped organ that stores about 50ml of bile until the body needs it for digestion. Bile is a bitter, yellow/green alkaline fluid secreted by hepacytes (special cells) in the liver. The human liver can produce close to one litre of bile per day.

The bile stored in the gallbladder is between 5-10 times more concentrated and potent that the bile secreted directly by the liver. This bile is discharged into the duodenum – the first part of the small intestine – mainly for the emulsification (breakdown) of fats during digestion. This is why people that have had their gallbladder removed are likely to have a tough time digesting fatty food.

The Relationship of the Gallbladder and Other Organs
Bile acts to some extent as a detergent, helping to emulsify fats (increasing surface area to help enzyme action), and thus aid in their absorption in the small intestine. The most important compounds are the salts of taurocholic acid and deoxycholic acid. Bile salts combine with phospholipids to break down fat globules in the process of emulsification by associating its hydrophobic side with lipids and the hydrophilic side with water.
Emulsified droplets are then organized into many micelles which increases absorption. Since bile increases the absorption of fats, it is an important part of the absorption of the fat-soluble vitamins D, E, K and A.

Besides its digestive function, bile serves as the route of excretion for the haemoglobin breakdown product (bilirubin) which gives bile its colour. It also neutralises any excess stomach acid before it enters the ileum, the final section of the small intestine. Bile salts are also bactericidal to the invading microbes that enter with food.

What is Bile?

The spleen breaks down worn-out red blood cells into bile salts and other substances. The liver removes excess bile salts and waste and sends them to the gallbladder for storage. The liver is the body's principal chemical plant - if you built a plant to perform all the chemical functions one person's liver could perform, the plant would cover *500 acres.*

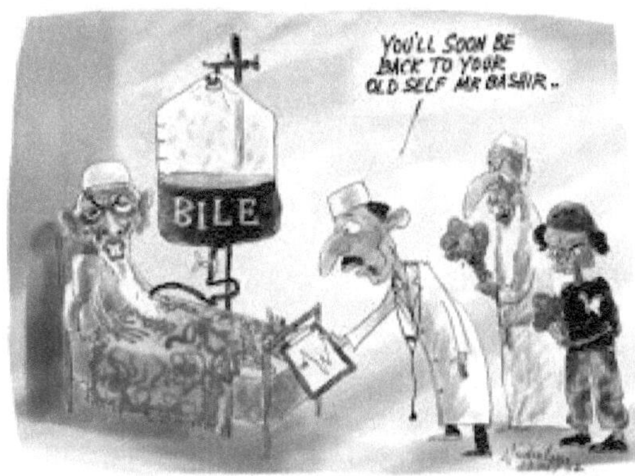

While the products are in the gallbladder, water is reabsorbed and so the waste products get more and more concentrated and form bile.

Bile is needed for 3 things:

1. As bile is very alkaline, it neutralizes the acid from the stomach
2. Bile breaks down fats so that they can be digested
3. Bile is a natural laxative for the colon.

Bile is essential in the digestion of fats. When you eat a meal with fats, the gallbladder releases a LARGE amount of bile to digest the fats. One big problem when a person has gallbladder surgery is that the body has nowhere to store bile until it is needed. Therefore, it just drips continually. When a fatty meal is eaten, there is simply not enough bile to digest the fat, causing indigestion on many occasions.

If the tubing or the ducts of the gallbladder are filled with gallstones, then this can cause a number of health problems including allergies or hives, but some have no symptoms at all. These stones cannot be seen by ultrasound scan or X-rays as they are not actually in the gallbladder but in the ducts; they may also not be calcified stones. There are many types of gallstones, most of which have cholesterol crystals in them. They can be black, red, white, green or tan coloured.

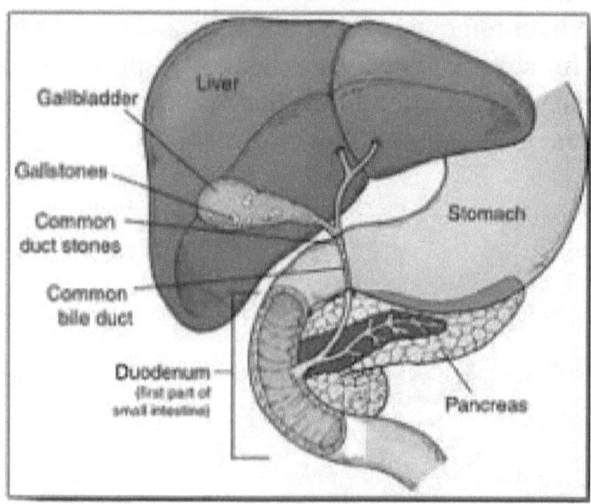

As the stones grow and become more numerous, the back pressure on the liver causes it to make less bile. It is also thought to slow the flow of lymphatic fluid. Imagine the situation if your garden hose had small stones in it – the result would be that much less water would flow. When there are gallstones, much less cholesterol leaves the body, resulting in elevated cholesterol levels.

Moreover, gallstones are porous so can pick up all the bacteria, cysts, viruses and parasites that are passing through the liver. These masses or "nests" of infectious material hang around the liver and supply the blood flowing through it with lots of fresh bugs daily. This is one way that parasites are circulated and reproduce.

These parasites and infectious nests must be removed, and the simplest way of doing that is to remove the gallstones.

How do we remove these gallstones without resorting to surgery?

Gallstones

Gallstones are a major cause of morbidity worldwide. In the United States, over 10% of the total population has gallstones. Each year 1,000,000 new patients are diagnosed. Performance of 500,000 cholecystectomies (gallbladder removal) leads to an annual expense of more than $5 billion in direct costs.

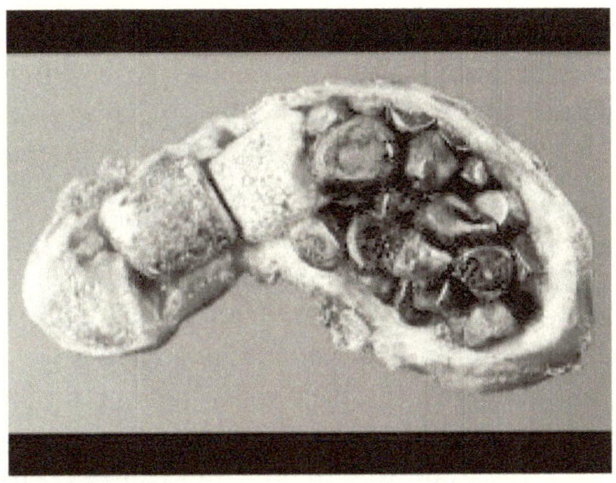

Pathogenesis of Gallstones

Gallstones are made mainly of cholesterol, bilirubin and calcium salts, with smaller amounts of protein and other materials. In Western countries, essentially all gallstones, whether cholesterol or pigmented, arise in the gallbladder. In Asia, a significant fraction of pigmented stones originates in the bile ducts. In Western countries cholesterol is the principal constituent of more than three quarters of gallstones.

In the simplest sense, cholesterol gallstones form when the cholesterol concentration in bile exceeds the ability of bile to hold cholesterol in solution. Non-cholesterol stones are categorized as black or brown pigment stones, consisting of calcium salts of bilirubin.

Most of the stones are made of cholesterol (75-80%), with bilirubin stones (also called black pigment stones) being far less and consisting of calcium bilirubinate, with large amounts of mucoprotein. Brown pigment stones are usually the hardest and smallest of the stones and these are usually made of calcium salts of unconjugated bilirubin, with variable amounts of protein and cholesterol.

How do I Know I have Gallstones?

I have personally seen many hundreds of patients who have undergone the liver and gallbladder cleanse under my supervision. Many of these patients who came for other problems, including chronic diseases, did not have any symptoms of gallbladder problems. However, nearly every single one of these flushed gallstones during the procedure.

Statistics tell us that about 80% of people harbouring gallstones are asymptomatic (have no symptoms) at any given point in time. Approximately 20% of these patients will become symptomatic over a 10-15-year period.

Symptoms and Signs of Gallbladder Problems

The following are some signs and indications showing the presence of gallstones in the liver and gallbladder. If you have any of them you are most likely to derive great benefits from having a liver cleanse and gallbladder cleanse. Generally, I would say that these markings are pretty accurate and play an important role in deciding whether a patient requires a gallbladder cleanse, even though everyone benefits in one way or other from these cleanses. Of course, the proof is in the pudding – the only way to prove that you have gallstones is to undergo the gallbladder flush and see the stones for yourself. The health benefits can also be enormous with many symptoms melting away literally overnight!

Let's look at some of the signs and symptoms that can present themselves when you have gallstones. This does not mean that everyone with gallstones will have all of these symptoms, but generally if you have gallstones you are expected to have some of these markings:

The Skin

The skin does not only react to external stimuli irritating it, it is also a barometer of the internal state of the body and can reflect the internal condition of tissues and organs.

This may show as skin blemishes, discoloration, or changed condition such as dryness, oiliness and wrinkles. In Traditional Chinese Medicine, there is a direct relationship between the skin and the liver. The following marks are particularly indicative of gallstones in the liver and gallbladder:

➤ ***Brown patches or Black spots*** – these usually look like freckles but are somewhat darker. These can be small (0.5 cm) or quite large (5+ cm). These can also be *moles* appearing on the right or left side of the forehead, between the eyebrows, under the eyes, and just above the right shoulder or between the shoulder blades.

Most prominent are the so-called *liver spots* on the back of the hands and forearms, often seen among middle-aged and elderly people. If gallstones that were excreted by the gall bladder get caught in the colon, such spots will appear in the area where the thumb and index finger meet. The liver spots and marks begin to fade after all stones are removed from the liver and gallbladder.

➤ ***A green or dark colour of the temple area at the sides of the head*** show that the liver, gallbladder, pancreas and spleen are underactive due to the deposits of gallstones in both the liver and gallbladder. This may be accompanied by a green or blue colour on both sides of the bridge of the nose, which indicates impaired spleen functions.

➤ ***Hair loss in the central region of the head*** indicates that the liver, heart, small intestines, pancreas, and reproductive organs are becoming increasingly congested and rigid. There is a tendency to develop cardiovascular disease, chronic digestive problems, and formation of cysts and tumours. *Grey and white hair* shows that the liver and gall bladder functions are underactive.

➤ ***An oily skin condition of the forehead*** also implies poor liver performance due to gallstones. So does *excessive perspiration* in this part of the head. *A yellow colour of the facial skin* indicates disorders of the bile functions of the liver and gallbladder, and a weakness of the pancreas, kidneys and excretory organs.

➤ ***Vertical wrinkles between the eyebrows***. There may be one deep line or two, sometimes three lines in this region. These wrinkles, which are *not* a part of natural ageing, indicate an accumulation of many gallstones in the liver. The liver is expanded and has hardened. The deeper and longer the wrinkles are, the more progressed the deterioration of liver function is. The vertical lines also represent a great deal of repressed frustration and anger. Anger arises when gallstones prevent proper bile flow. If white or yellow patches accompany the wrinkles, there may be a cyst or tumour developing in the liver. Pimples or growth of hair between the eyebrows, with or without wrinkles, indicate that the liver, gallbladder and spleen are affected.

> ➢ ***Horizontal wrinkles across the bridge of the nose*** are a sign of pancreatic disorders due to gallstones in the liver. If a line is very deep and pronounced, there may be *pancreatitis* or *diabetes*.

The Nose

The nose is not only used for smelling and blowing – it is another correspondence system that can help us understand our internal state. Here are some signs related to the gallbladder and liver:

> ➢ ***A red colour of the nose*** shows an abnormal condition of the heart, with tendency towards hypertension. A purple nose indicates low blood pressure. Both conditions are caused by imbalanced liver functions.

> ➢ ***A nose bending towards the left*** indicates that the organs on the right-hand side of the body – including the liver, gall bladder, right kidney, ascending colon, right ovary or testicle - are underactive. The main cause for this condition is an accumulation of gallstones in the liver and gallbladder (the nose will return to centre when the stones   are   removed).

The Eyes

Again, the eyes are also another excellent correspondence system that has connections to many different body systems. The study of Iridology can help to identify many different issues in the body. Here we are not looking at the eye under an iris microscope, but with the naked eye.

> ➢ ***A yellowish colour of the skin under the eyes*** indicates that the liver and gallbladder are overactive. A dark colour arises when the kidneys, bladder, and reproductive organs are overtaxed as a result

of a long-standing disorder of the digestive functions.

> ➤ ***White/yellow fatty deposits on the white of the eye, usually found either side of the pupil*** show that the body is accumulating fatty substances; the liver and gallbladder functions are impaired. If these patches are white in colour, this is indicative of large amounts of cholesterol having accumulated in the circulatory and lymphatic system.

The Tongue

If you have been to a Chinese Medicine doctor you will know that they use the tongue a lot in diagnosing a whole bunch of health problems. What a simple and beautiful way of "talking" to your body.

> ➤ ***The tongue is coated yellow/white, especially in its back part.*** This indicates an imbalance in the secretion of bile, which is the major cause of digestive trouble.

> ➤ ***Cracks on the tongue*** are signs of impaired colon function. Food is not mixed sufficiently with bile and which permits toxic acids to injure and derange the colon walls. There may be little or no mucous discharge on the tongue.

> ➤ ***Repeated mucous discharge into the throat and mouth.*** Bile may regurgitate into the stomach, which irritates its protective lining and causes excessive mucus production. Some of the bile and mucus may even move up towards the mouth. This may create a bad taste (bitter) in the mouth and give rise to frequent attempts of clearing the throat which involves coughing.

> ➤ ***The lips become dark in places*** when obstructions in the liver, gall bladder and kidneys have resulted in slowness and stagnation of blood circulation and lymph drainage throughout the body. There may be advanced abnormal constriction of blood capillaries. If the colour becomes reddish, the heart, lungs and respiratory functions are subdued.

> ***Teeth problems*** in general are related to poor liver function. Tooth decay in particular is caused by nutritional imbalance. Poor digestion and overconsumption of refined, processed and highly acid-forming foods such as sugar, chocolate, meat, cheese, coffee and soda pops deplete minerals and vitamins. Adults usually have 32 teeth. Each tooth corresponds to one of the 32 vertebrae of the spine and each vertebra is connected to a major organ or gland. If any of the 4 canines are decaying, it indicates the presence of large numbers of gallstones in the liver and gallbladder. A yellow colour of the teeth and the canines may indicate disorders in all the mid-abdominal region, i.e. the liver, gallbladder, stomach, pancreas, spleen and their functions.

The Hands and Feet

You are all probably aware of reflexology - a method of analysing and treating through the soles of the feet that correspond to the rest of the body. The hand is also another excellent correspondence organ that can give much information about the whole body – this is used in *Su Jok* Acupuncture, a Korean form of acupuncture.

Imagine that you have a whole "clinic" on your hands and feet that corresponds to your whole body.

> ***White, fatty skin on the fingertips*** indicates disorders of the digestive and lymphatic systems and the liver and kidneys may be forming cysts and tumours. There is discharge of excessive fats and sugar.

> ***Dark red fingernails*** show a high content of cholesterol, fatty acids, and minerals in the blood. The liver, gallbladder and spleen are congested and underactive and all excretory functions are overloaded.

> ***Whitish nails*** indicate accumulation of fat and mucus in and around the heart, liver, pancreas, prostate and ovaries.

➢ ***Vertical ridges on the nails*** generally indicate poor absorption of food and disruption of digestive, liver and kidney functions.

➢ ***Hard protrusion at the ball of the foot.*** This condition shows progressive hardening of the organs in the middle of the body, including the liver, stomach, pancreas, and spleen. There are numerous gallstones in the liver and gallbladder.

➢ ***A yellow colour of the feet*** also indicates an accumulation of many stones in the liver and gallbladder. If the colour becomes green, the spleen and lymph functions are severely disrupted which may lead to cysts, tumours and cancer.

➢ ***Hardness at the tip of the fourth toe or a callous in the area under the fourth toe*** is an indication that gallbladder functions are stagnant. General rigidity, bent condition, and painful fourth toes show that there is a history of gallstones in the gall bladder and liver.

➢ ***Curving of the first toe.*** If the large (first) toe curves abnormally, i.e. towards the second toe, it shows that the liver functions are subdued due to the presence of gallstones in the liver bile ducts. At the same time, spleen and lymphatic functions are overactive due to the accumulation of toxic residues from inadequately digested foods.

➢ ***A white colour and rugged surfaces on the fourth and fifth toenails*** indicate disorders in the liver and gallbladder as well as the kidneys and bladder.

The Constitution of Faecal Matter
As unpleasant as this may be, you can elicit a lot of health information by looking at your stools. The texture and smell of the stool is very indicative of internal body functioning.

➢ ***The faeces look pale or clay-coloured*** is an indication of poor liver performance (bile gives the stool its natural brown colour). If it floats, large amounts of undigested fats are contained in it, which makes it lighter than water.

Conclusion

There may be many more signs and marks indicating the presence of gallstones in the liver and gall bladder than those listed above. For example, pain in the right shoulder, tennis elbow, frozen shoulder, numbness in the legs, sciatica, all may have no obvious relation to gallstones that have accumulated in the liver, yet by removing the gallstones, these conditions disappear.

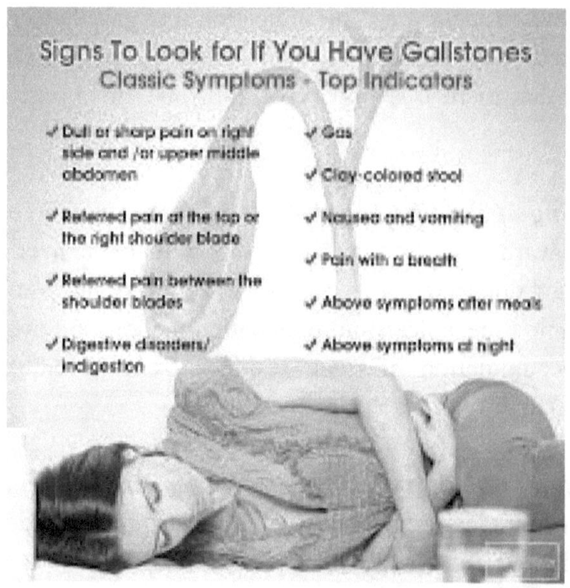

13

CHAPTER 2:

WHAT ARE TOXINS?

A toxin is anything that is harmful or detrimental to the body.
Toxins can be internal (created by the biological processes of the body) or external (something that is introduced to the body, ingested, absorbed or inhaled).

The immune system, gastrointestinal (GI) system and skin are designed to protect you from toxins. However, you are exposed to toxic substances daily via what you apply to your skin, what you breathe and what you ingest.

Within your lifetime, you will consume up to 50 tonnes of food. Your GI system is responsible for breaking down these foods, digesting and absorbing components which are useful and eliminating the rest.

The liver works to remove toxins from the food you eat as well as toxins produced by your body. When the GI tract is not functioning well, the liver must do more work due to the additional burden placed upon it.

What Do Toxins Do to the Body?
When toxins build up, the ability for your body to remove them is quickly impaired. The body's self-regulation systems go out of balance, digestion becomes impaired and the liver and immune system become overwhelmed and cannot keep up.

The function of the large intestine slows down which in turn leads to congestion in the lymphatic system - which is designed to drain waste products from blood and tissues - thus forcing waste to re-circulate within the body.

When the liver is clogged, it allows toxins to travel into the body, instead of filtering them out. Toxins then get into the bloodstream and cause inflammation in other parts of the body. Thus, the body resorts to using the skin to purge the waste. Acne, rashes and eczema are signs that the body is trying to rid itself of toxins.

Toxins are also stored in body fat, causing weight gain and preventing the body from fully detoxifying itself.

How Do You Know That You are Toxic?
Do you suffer from tiredness, lethargy, a 'heavy' feeling, digestive problems, bowel distension, headaches, muscle aches, poor concentration and memory, insomnia and many other symptoms too numerous to list? Well, all these symptoms can be related to toxins in your body that have accumulated over time.

Table 1 below shows some common signs and symptoms of toxicity:

Headaches	Backache	Runny nose	Fatigue
Joint pains	Itchy nose	Nervousness	Skin rashes
Cough	Frequent colds	Sleepiness	Hives
Wheezing	Irritated eyes	Insomnia	Nausea
Sore throat	Immune weakness	Dizziness	Indigestion
Tight or stiff neck	Environmental sensitivity	Mood changes	Anorexia
Angina Pectoris	Sinus congestion	Anxiety	Bad breath
Circulatory deficits	Fever	Depression	Constipation
High blood fats	Unexplained irritability	Chronic fatigue	Muscle twitching

Table 1. Signs and symptoms of toxicity

Signs and Symptoms of Toxicity
Life is toxic! There are toxins in the food you eat, the water you drink and the air you breathe. Even your own body produces toxins as a result of its many metabolic processes that keep you alive.

Signs that detoxification is needed if you have:

- ❖ Unexplained headaches or back pain
- ❖ Joint pain or arthritis
- ❖ Memory failure
- ❖ Depression or lack of energy
- ❖ Brittle nails and hair

❖ Abnormal body odour, coated tongue or bad breath
❖ Unexplained weight gain
❖ Psoriasis
❖ Frequent allergies
❖ A history of heavy alcohol use
❖ A history of natural and synthetic steroid hormone use
❖ An exposure to cleaning solvents, pesticides, diuretics and certain drugs.

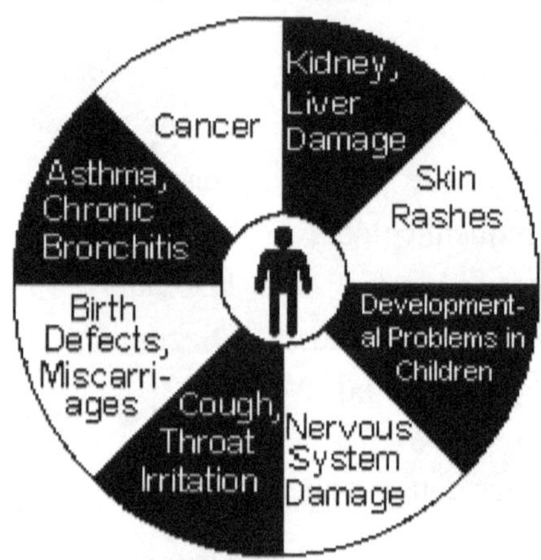

Benefits of Detoxification
There are several benefits of detoxification such as:

❖ The digestive tract is cleansed of accumulated waste and fermenting bacteria.
❖ Liver, kidney and blood purification can take place, which is not possible during regular eating patterns.
❖ Mental clarity is enhanced as chemical and food additive overload is reduced.
❖ Reduced dependency on habit-forming substances such as sugar, caffeine, nicotine, alcohol and drugs.
❖ The stomach size is returned to normal as bad eating habits are stopped.
❖ The hormonal system is enhanced which is especially true for growth hormones.
❖ The immune system is stimulated.

It never ceases to amaze me that most symptoms, if not all, can disappear in less than 15 days! After detoxifying on an alkaline diet for 15 days, patients report high energy levels; clear and glowing skin with a brilliance that is obvious (I have said on many occasions that I should take before-detox and after-detox photos of patients - the change is striking!); weight loss of several pounds, which is an excellent motivating factor to continue with a detox programme; clear-headedness; higher thresholds for stress and tension; reduced cellulite; good body tone and a great feeling of being relaxed.

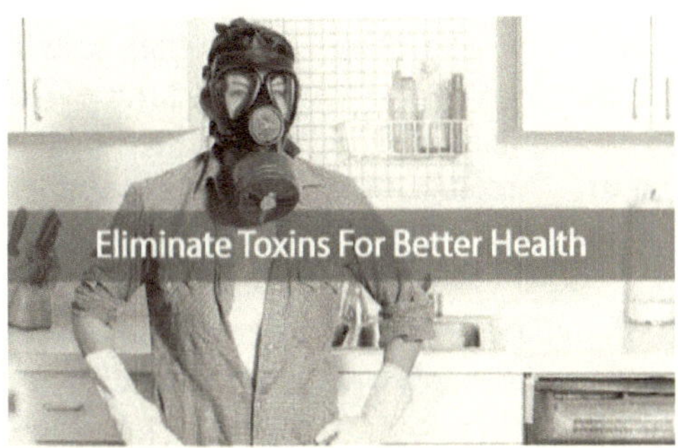

"How do you achieve this?" you may ask. Well, the secret lies in using a variety of detoxification protocols, which I will share with you later.

Detoxification has become a household word and a colloquialism that could mean anything from drinking a glass of carrot juice to entering a detoxification centre if you are an alcoholic or drug addict.

The term has now become a misnomer for many things that it is not. In the context that we are using the term, detoxification is the process of removing the toxins that have been accumulating in the body tissues and organs throughout a person's life. These toxins will have been acting as metabolism blockers by literally poisoning the cells and not allowing them to function correctly.

You can have toxins stored in your body for years without experiencing any negative symptoms. It is only when the toxin levels become too high that you start to feel ill.

Sources of Toxins
So where do toxins come from? There are many sources, some of which I will mention here.

The three main sources are:

a) <u>Exogenous toxins</u>:
Exogenous toxins (Greek: 'from outside') are those that enter our bodies from the outside, i.e. food additives, pesticides, herbicides, fungi from food, industrial pollutants, viruses, bacteria, parasites and electromagnetic pollution such as X-rays, electromagnetic radiation and geopathic stress.

These external toxins may also come from other sources such as water, beverages, alcohol, medicines, accidents and injuries. Various industries have polluted our environment with an array of toxic heavy metals such as aluminium, antimony, arsenic, beryllium, bismuth, cadmium, lead, mercury, nickel, thallium and uranium.

Bisphenol A and Phthalates, commonly referred to as BPA, are toxic substances that exist in cheap plastic drinking bottles. While most bottles with BPA have been phased out, some still use them and should be avoided. A 2015 study confirmed that about 44% of canned food producers still use BPA-lined cans.

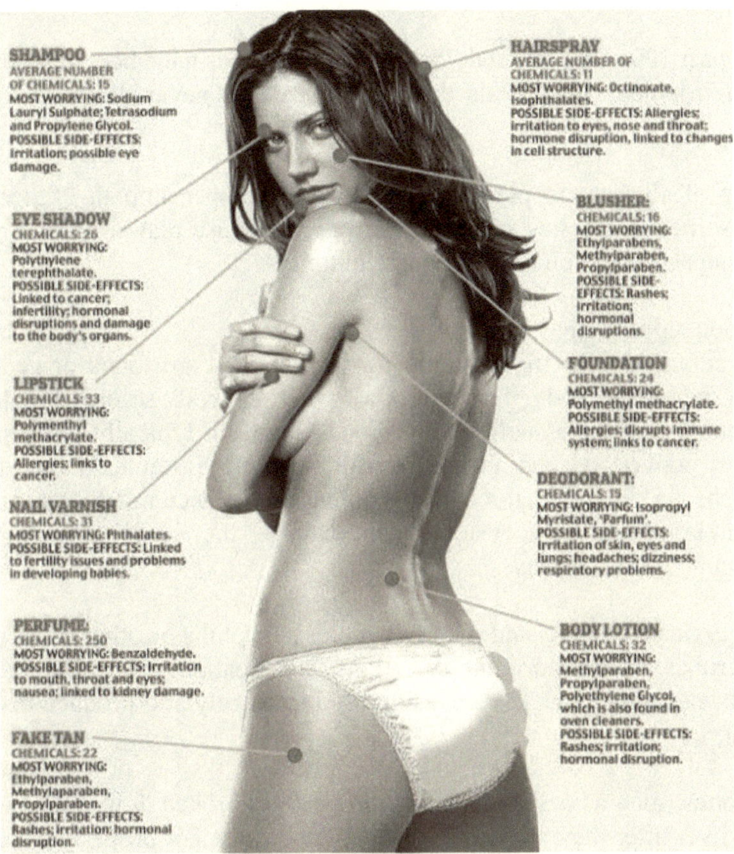

Amalgam teeth fillings contain 50% mercury, which is a potent neurotoxin. We will discuss this later when we talk about toxicity and heavy metals.

Processed foods contain artificial food additives, colours, flavours and preservatives.

Meat often contains hormones and antibiotics, which can cause hormonal disruption.

Caffeine and other stimulants, sedatives, alcohol, tobacco and illegal drugs, all must be filtered out of the body through the liver and kidneys.

Household chemicals are also guilty of introducing toxins into indoor living spaces. Common surface cleaners can emit dangerous fumes that may concentrate in small, enclosed areas. Even pet products may contain toxic elements that can harm both you and your pet.

In the past 100 years, around 75,000 new chemicals have been released into the environment. Chemicals that your body was never designed to cope with.

On top of all that, people are not getting the proper amount of sleep and exercise needed to stay healthy. Sleep and exercise play a critical role in relieving stress and eliminating harmful toxins.

b) <u>Endogenous toxins</u>:
Endogenous (Greek: 'from within') are toxins that are found or generated within the human body. This can occur when the body's normal metabolic mechanisms function inefficiently. For example, it typically takes several steps to convert the amino acid methionine into cysteine. If one step is sluggish, an intermediate called homocysteine accumulates in tissues. Accumulation of homocysteine can damage the vascular system and contribute to heart disease.[1]

Other toxins are associated with tuberculosis, syphilis or other diseases due to microbes; excess hormone secretions; constipation, producing toxins in the gut; pathogenic bacteria, causing food to putrefy and produce toxins in the gut;[2].

Hormones, such as oestrogen and androgen, get broken down and excreted in the liver after they are used. If the hormones are not properly taken care of by the liver, then hormonal imbalances and symptoms occur. Toxic build-up can occur when elimination mechanisms are inadequate due to poor nutrient intake or malabsorption of key detoxification nutrients.

Emotional stress is also a large contributor to toxins in the body. Research has shown that there is a connection between your emotions and well-being. When experiencing a traumatic or stressful event, it is

common to react with anger, fear, grief, resentment etc. Repeated cycles of emotional stresses have a direct effect on the nervous and hormonal systems, which can indirectly affect our body's ability to detoxify.

---

[1] Graham, I, Daly, L, Refsum H, et al. Plasma homocysteine as a risk factor for vascular disease. *JAMA*. 277;1775-1781, 1997.
[2] Donovan P. Bowel toxemia, permeability and disease: new information to support an old concept. In: Pizzorno JE, Murray MT. Textbook of Natural Medicine. St. Louis, MO: Elsevier Ltd; 1993.

Not dealing with your issues, and the emotions that get triggered by them, does not make the issue go away and only adds to the damaging effects on the body.

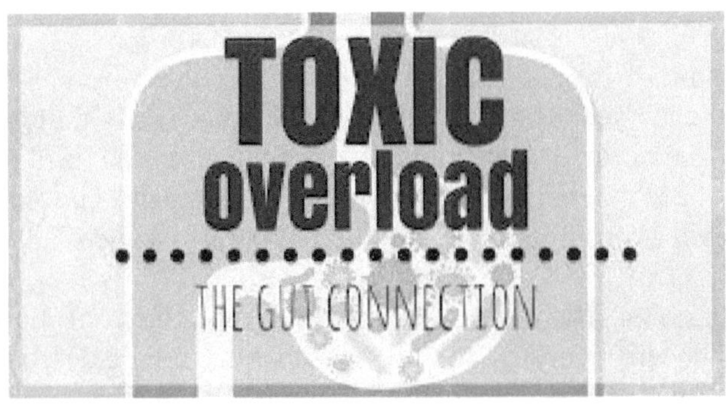

c) <u>Autogenous toxins</u>:

Autogenous toxins (Greek: 'Born within') are generated within the body from miasmic influences, which are inherited tendencies that can pass through up to seven generations. Examples of these are psora, sycosis, tuberculosis, syphilinum and others. There is no detection of these pathogens with scientific testing, but their deep presence can affect the body's organs, primarily by inhibiting a good immune response and lowering its resistance.

Let's look at some specific sources of toxins that we encounter daily:

Cigarettes, alcohol, caffeine and drugs are all substances that the body cannot use for building and repair, so will add to the mounting waste. A lot of these toxic wastes are stored in the tissues and organs of the body.

Heavy metals such as mercury from fish and amalgam fillings; aluminium found in cheeses, baking powders, cake mixes, self-raising flour, cosmetics, toothpastes, antiperspirants and some drugs such as antacids. Cadmium is found in tea and coffee, as well as cigarette smoke. Lead is found in paints, fuels, rubber, plastics, inks, dyes, toys, building materials and hair restorers.

Arsenic is given to chickens as a growth promoter. Roxarsone - 4-hydroxy-3-nitrobenzenearsonic acid - is by far the most common arsenic-based additive used in chicken feed.[3] It is mixed in the diet of about 70% of the 9 billion broiler chickens produced annually in the U.S. In its original organic form, roxarsone is relatively benign. It is less toxic than the inorganic forms of arsenic-arsenite.

However, some of the 2.2 million lbs of roxarsone mixed in the nation's chicken feed each year converts into inorganic arsenic within the bird, and the rest is transformed into inorganic forms after the bird excretes it. Arsenic has been linked to bladder, lung, skin, kidney and colon cancer, while low-level exposures can lead to partial paralysis and diabetes.

Plastics containing Bisphenol A, the building block of polycarbonate plastics, which are everywhere: in pesticides as fungicides, antioxidants, flame retardants, rubber chemicals, a coating in metals, cans and food containers, refrigerator shelving, returnable containers for juice, milk and water, nail polish, compact discs, adhesives, microwave ovenware and eating utensils.

A diet that is high in animal fats will add to the waste. There are many different drugs and chemicals that are given to animals these days, ranging from antibiotics, hormones, feed concentrates, etc. All these chemicals will accumulate in the fat cells of the animals that we then eat – so we slowly build up an accumulation of these chemicals over time.

Sluggish bowels can lead to a great deal of toxicity throughout the body.

Try to imagine a 10-metre tube running from mouth to anus packed with meat, sausage, fish, fruit salad, beef burgers, sugars, milk and other goodies – all fermenting and putrefying for days on end.

This fermentation produces highly toxic substances such as putrescine, neuracine and cadaverine. These are so poisonous that a small amount injected into a laboratory animal will kill it in minutes. All these toxic substances, apart from causing disease in the body, will also act as metabolism blockers, and will therefore have consequences on weight-loss too.

---

[3] Hileman, B. Arsenic in Chicken Production: A common feed additive adds arsenic to human food and endangers water supplies. *Chemical and Engineering News.* Volume 85, Number 15, pp. 34-35, April 9, 2007.

This process of 'self-poisoning' by these putrefying foods in the gut is called 'autointoxication.'

Refined foods such as white sugar, white flour, white rice, etc. are all deficient in nutrients, but calorie loaded. Apart from this, they also help to create a lot of sludge and debris in the body. If you remember from your childhood days, you probably used white flour and water to make a glue to make your kite, or to glue your coloured paper in your exercise book at school.

When eaten, white flour and its products become glue in the intestine and stick to the internal walls. When mixed with sticky sugar and fat, it becomes a rubber-like substance that blocks absorption of foods through the intestine, as well as being a constant source of toxins. If you don't believe me, read Dr. Jensen's book entitled, *'Tissue cleansing through bowel management'*[4]. There are also plenty of photos of what actually comes out of the intestine if you do a proper detox – disgusting!

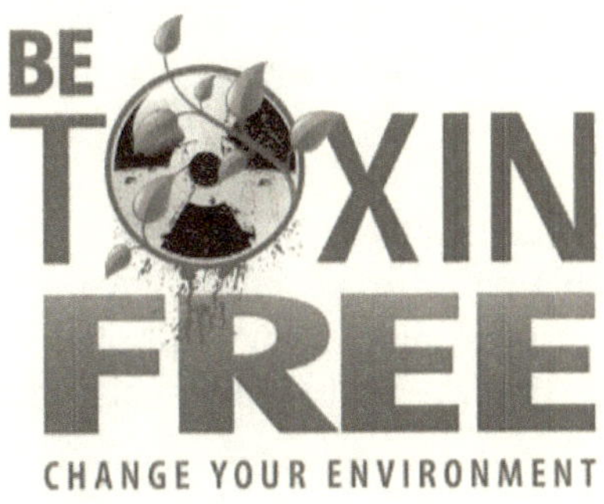

Thousands of new, toxic chemical compounds are produced each year by the chemical industry, most of which are approved by various so-called 'Environmental Protection Agencies' (EPA's) without any serious toxicological studies. The cumulative number of toxic chemicals polluting our planet today exceeds 100,000.

Many claim that some of these chemicals, such as the flame retardants used in children's clothing, have potentially life-saving applications. But how

---

[4] Jensen, B. Dr. Jensen's guide to better bowel care: A complete program for tissue cleansing through bowel management. USA: Avery Publishers, 1999.

many of these chemicals do we ingest or are absorbed by our bodies and those of our children? And at what cost to our health? What is the capacity of the human body to eliminate them?

Has anyone conducted a general contracting cost-benefit analysis as to whether the benefits offered, for example, by fire hazard protection, truly outweigh the toxicity generated within us, our children and the environment? The answer is: *No*. There are no comprehensive, scientific answers, other than to confirm the obvious: toxicity levels in humans and animals across the globe are rising fast. Whether we realize it or not – *we are all toxic*.

In an article published in the October 2006 *National Geographic* entitled, *'The Pollution Within,'* journalist David Ewing Duncan had himself tested for 320 synthetic chemicals and certain heavy metals at a cost of $16,000, paid for by the magazine.

According to the article, Duncan was considered a healthy individual. Nevertheless, he had higher than average amounts of chemical toxins, such as flame-retardants (known as PDBE's), phthalates, Polychlorinated Biphenyls (PCBs), pesticides and dioxins, as well as heavy metals such as mercury.

Duncan's article alludes to some of the possible ways toxic chemicals may have accumulated in his body: some might have originated in childhood, while others may have been picked up in airplanes due to his extensive work-related travel. However, he and his doctors were merely speculating…

Duncan also describes his pre- and post-mercury toxicity results after a fresh fish dinner and breakfast. Duncan had fresh halibut for dinner and fresh swordfish for breakfast (cooked in his toxic non-stick pan), both of which were caught in the ocean just outside the Golden Gate Bridge in the San Francisco Bay area.

He tested himself for serum mercury before and after the meals, and found that his blood mercury levels had shot up from five micrograms per litre to over 12. The doctors conducting the tests advised him not to repeat that experiment ever again, yet I'm sure this dangerous diet is adhered to by thousands, unaware of the impact of toxicity on their health. After all, fish is promoted as a health food! Nevertheless, drawing conclusions on the experience of only one healthy adult is not robust, toxicological science. So, let us review the research.

New 21st Century Theory of Disease
Dr. Miller, of the Department of Family Practice, University of Texas Health Science Center at San Antonio, USA, believes that we are on the threshold of the new theory of disease that is triggered by toxic chemicals. She states in one of her papers[5]:

"In the late 1800's, physicians observed that certain illnesses spread from sick, feverish individuals to those contacting them, paving the way for the germ theory of disease. The germ theory served as a crude but elegant formulation that explained dozens of seemingly unrelated illnesses affecting literally every organ system."

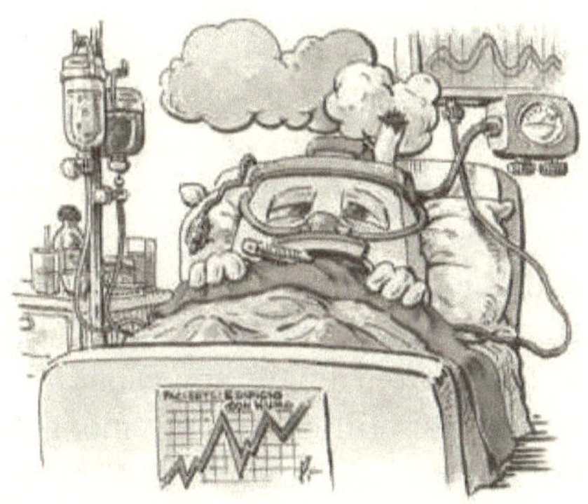

She continues:

"Today we are witnessing another medical anomaly – the unique pattern of illness involving chemically exposed people who subsequently report multisystem symptoms and new-onset chemical and food intolerances. These intolerances may be the hallmark for a new disease process, just as fever is a hallmark for infection."

---

[5] Miller C. Are We on the Threshold of a New Theory of Disease? Toxicant-induced Loss of Tolerance and its Relationship to Addiction and Abdiction. *Tox. Ind. Health.* 15:284-294, 1999.

I strongly agree with Dr Miller and believe that many of the new diseases that we are seeing today such as Gulf War Syndrome,[6] Chronic Fatigue Syndrome, Myalgic Encephalomyelitis (ME), fibromyalgia, childhood diabetes, attention deficit hyperactivity disorder and others are all chemically related disorders.[7]

How exposed are you to these chemicals?
Check out below how prone you are to develop a chemically-triggered 21st century disease, by checking off the various categories. The more of these that apply to you, the higher your risk. Do you:

- ✓ Work with chemicals
- ✓ Use pesticides around the house and garden such as fly spray, weed killer or flea powder
- ✓ Use non-environmentally friendly cosmetics, toiletries and household cleaners
- ✓ You are responsible for disposal of chemicals used in medicines such as mercury preservatives in vaccines and flea shampoo
- ✓ Eat nonorganic fruit, vegetables and meat products
- ✓ Eat contaminated seafood, usually containing mercury
- ✓ Eat too many processed foods, full of preservatives, colourings, flavourings and other additives
- ✓ Drink unfiltered tap water containing aluminium and fluoride
- ✓ Consume soft drinks from aluminium cans
- ✓ Have mercury amalgam fillings in your mouth
- ✓ Live in a major city with all the air pollution.

---

[6] Miller, C. and Prihoda, TA Controlled Comparison of Symptoms and Chemical Intolerances Reported by Gulf War Veterans, Implant Recipients and Persons with Multiple Chemical Sensitivity. *Tox. Ind. Health* 15:386-397, 1999.
[7] Miller, C. Prihoda, T. The Environmental Exposure and Sensitivity Inventory (EESI): A Standardized approach for measuring Chemical Intolerances for Research and Clinical Applications. *Tox. Ind. Health* 15:370-385, 1999.

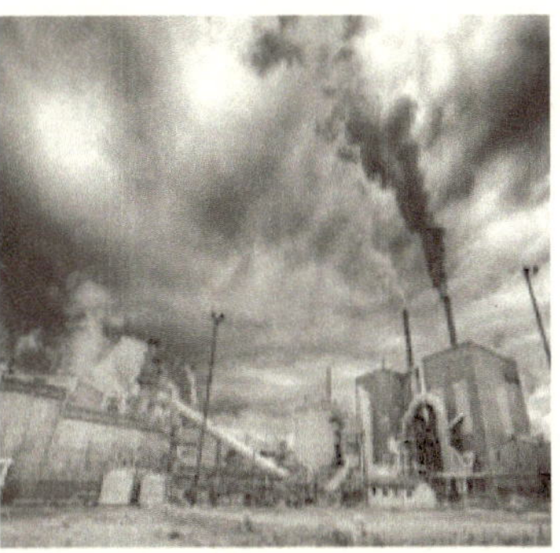

These chemicals are accumulative, so do not think that a little exposure will do you no harm – it simply takes longer to reach critical levels in the body before symptoms appear.

Signs and Symptoms of Chemical Poisoning

In clinical practice, I am often very vigilant in trying to detect symptoms that are related to chemical sensitivity and other toxicity issues. If the patient suddenly develops the following symptoms, then chemical exposure should be suspected:

- ✓ Dark blue, black or pink circles under the eyes
- ✓ Wrinkles or abnormally puffy bags under the eyes, as well as wrinkles on hands and knuckles
- ✓ Bright red cheeks, nose tips or ear lobes
- ✓ Unstable legs
- ✓ A spaced-out look and feeling
- ✓ Itchy nose
- ✓ Licking lips frequently
- ✓ Fuzzy thinking, confusion; difficulty in concentrating, thinking clearly or remembering
- ✓ Joint or arthritic pains
- ✓ Runny nose or nasal congestion causing sinusitis and blocked nose
- ✓ Extreme fatigue, even when rising in the morning
- ✓ Headaches

One study that tried to assess exposure to Bisphenol A (BPA) and 4-tertiary-octylphenol (tOP) in the American population found 92.6% and 57.4% of the persons, respectively had these chemicals in their urine.[8]

These are industrial chemicals used in the manufacture of polycarbonate plastics and epoxy resins (BPA) and non-ionic surfactants (tOP). These products are in widespread use in the United States and the rest of the world.

Disorders Linked to Heavy Metal Toxicity		
Attention Deficit Disorder	Parkinson's disease	Asthma
Autism Spectrum disorders	Thyroid disorders	Arthritis
Auto-immune disorders	Multiple Scleroris	Candidiasis
Chronic Fatigue Syndrome	Kidney disease	Epilepsy
Lou Gehrig's disease (ALS)	Schizophrenia	Fibromyalgia
Gulf War Syndrome	Hypertension	Insomnia
Alzheimer's disease	Liver disease	Infertility

Ways to Address Toxicity: The good, the bad and the ugly
Let's start with the ugly first: the typical misguided response to the toxicity onslaught is to visit the average doctor, who will note a few toxicity-induced symptoms, and come up with a superficial diagnosis.

At first, a diagnosis appears simple: flu, sinusitis, eczema, tonsillitis, or otitis. Over time, diagnoses get complicated: asthma, arthritis, sacroiliatis, heart disease, renal disease, liver disease, cancer or any of the currently labelled chronic degenerative diseases which can strike.
This ugly, symptom-based approach amounts to a classically wrong diagnosis.

The main causative factor, TOXICITY, remains undetected. Hardly anyone is searching for it, let alone finding it! Tragically, the ugly approach has become the norm, instead of the exception. Depending on the wrong diagnosis, which is typically a mere description of the symptom, the typical physician will prescribe chemical drugs to ingest, or refer you to other specialists who may contemplate removal of body parts (pardon the cynicism here, but this is the truth, as I experienced it from allopathic doctors – hopefully there will always be the exception among such practitioners).

---

[8] Calafat AM, Ye X, Wong LY, Reidy JA, Needham LL. Exposure of the U.S. Population to Bisphenol A and 4-*tertiary*-Octylphenol: 2003-2004. *Environ Health Perspect* Jan;116(1):39-44, 2008.

With the ugly approach, the worse the disease, the worse the treatment gets. Cancer, the dreaded disease, is the perfect example.

The reasoning goes: many toxins are proven carcinogens, so they could well be the cause of a person's cancer, right? Wrong! The ugly approach sees the world differently. Even at this advanced stage of body toxicity, when the body's immunity and vitality has been seriously compromised by carcinogens, the default medical intervention is to load the body with even more toxins: potent chemotherapeutic agents that are super-toxic, or cancer-causing radiation treatments to remove the original cancer.

You also need additional drugs (Erythropoietin Stimulating Agents) to counter the decrease in red blood cell production caused by chemotherapy, which add their own serious side-effects. By then, the tumour is reduced, the cancer has metastasized and the patient is either dead or bankrupt – or likely both. 'Common sense' at its best!

What we should be doing, medics and patients alike, is exactly the opposite. Should we not be addressing the cause of the problem - the toxins - instead of chasing and suppressing the symptoms? We should be reducing the toxic load, not increasing it.

We should be improving the tissue integrity, not cutting it apart. It seems evident to me that the common-sense approach would dictate addressing the safe removal of the toxins. Assuming our interest lies in achieving real, long-term relief for the patient.

Indeed, between the ugly and the good approach, there is also a bad way to address toxicity-caused illnesses.

If you try to release toxins from the body too fast, or too clumsily, the body may be tipped over the edge. This is an issue that many well-meaning practitioners underestimate – either because of inadequate technical know-how, insufficient experience or poor judgment – with disastrous results vis-à-vis the recovery prospects of their patients.

Unfortunately, there are plenty of bad ways out there to deal with toxicity-induced diseases. Therefore, sound and continuous research by the patient and practitioners to minimize such a risk is integral.

Meanwhile, a growing group of medical practitioners have 'jumped on the bandwagon' so to speak, using their medical licenses to chelate people with various heavy metals – using more drugs such as EDTA, DMSA, DMPS and the like. This can often lead to disastrous consequences as these drugs mobilize metals quicker than the body can eliminate them, while stripping the body of the good minerals.

SYMPTOMS OF TOXICITY

▪ Loss of energy	▪ Nausea	▪ Body aches and pains
▪ Memory loss	▪ Insomnia	▪ Frequent Headaches
▪ Depression	▪ Allergies	▪ Muscle stiffness
▪ Anxiety	▪ Nervousness	▪ Frequent colds
▪ Restlessness	▪ Skin irritation	▪ "Cold spots" sensation
▪ Mental Fog	▪ Food intolerance	▪ Deteriorating vision

In other words, the typical MD's knowledge of toxicology needs improvement, to say the least. There are natural, gentler ways of detoxifying the body of heavy metals and other xenobiotics.

I hope that this book, based on extensive research, will provide food-for-thought to the many out there that are lost and confused about these complex issues.

There is no doubt that the liver is the largest and most complex organ involved in the detoxification of the whole body. It may be worth spending a little time trying to understand the liver function in simple language.

Liver Structure and Function
There is no doubt that the liver is the largest and most complex organ involved in the detoxification of the whole body. It may be worth spending a little time trying to understand the liver function in simple language.

The characteristic structure and organization of the liver enables it to perform vital roles in regulating, synthesizing, storing, secreting, transforming, and breaking down many different substances in the body. In addition, the liver's ability to regenerate lost tissue helps maintain these functions, even in the face of moderate damage.

Functions of the Liver
The liver is the largest organ of the body with a diameter of about 20cm, a height of about 15cm and a depth of about 10cm. It weighs about 1,400

grams which is nearly 1.5 kilos or about 3.5 pounds – quite a chunky piece of meat as you can see from the photo of the calf liver below:

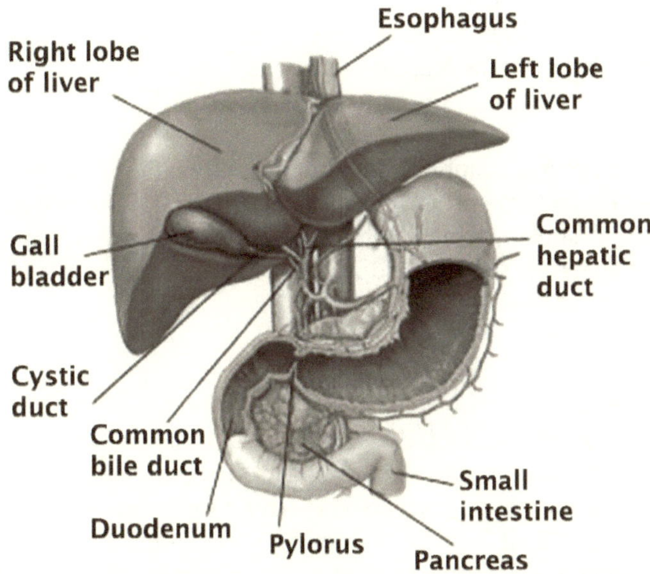

The liver has many different functions:

- It is responsible for the production of bile which is stored in the gallbladder and released when required for the digestion of fats.

- The liver stores glucose in the form of glycogen which is converted back to glucose again when needed for energy.

- It stores the vitamins A, D, K, B12 and folate and synthesizes blood clotting factors.

- Another important role is as a detoxifier, breaking down or transforming substances like ammonia, metabolic waste, drugs, alcohol and chemicals, so that they can be excreted.

These may also be referred to as "xenobiotic" chemicals. If we examine the liver under a microscope, we will see rows of liver cells separated by spaces which act like a filter or sieve, through which the blood stream flows. The liver filter is designed to remove toxic matter such as dead cells, microorganisms, chemicals, drugs and particulate debris from the blood stream. The liver filter is called the sinusoidal system, and contains specialized cells known as Kupffer cells which ingest and breakdown toxic matter.

Apart from removing xenobiotics and other toxins, the liver can remove a wide range of microorganisms such as bacteria, fungi, viruses and parasites from the blood stream, which is highly desirable, as we certainly do not want these dangerous things building up in the blood stream and invading the deeper parts of the body.

Toxic Overload
If the phase one and two detoxification pathways become overloaded, there will be a build-up of toxins in the body. Many of these toxins are fat soluble and incorporate themselves into fatty parts of the body where they may stay for years, if not for a lifetime. The brain and the endocrine (hormonal) glands are fatty organs and are common sites for fat-soluble toxins to accumulate. This may result in symptoms of brain dysfunction and hormonal imbalances, such as infertility, breast pain, menstrual disturbances, adrenal gland exhaustion and early menopause. Many of these chemicals (e.g. pesticides, petrochemicals) are carcinogenic and have been implicated in the rising incidence of many cancers.

Liver Symptoms
When there is toxic overload, certain symptoms develop which we will look at in more detail:

1. **Abnormal Metabolism of Fats**

    - Abnormalities in the level of fats in the blood stream, for example, elevated LDL cholesterol and reduced HDL cholesterol and elevated triglycerides
    - Arteries blocked with fat, leading to high blood pressure, heart attacks and strokes

- Build-up of fat in other body organs (fatty degeneration of organs)
- Lumps of fat in the skin (lipomas and other fatty tumours)
- Excessive weight gain, which may lead to obesity
- Inability to lose weight even while dieting
- Sluggish metabolism
- Protuberant abdomen (pot belly)
- Cellulite; fatty liver; roll of fat around the upper abdomen (liver roll)

2. **Digestive Problems**

- Indigestion
- Reflux
- Haemorrhoids
- Gall stones and gallbladder disease
- Intolerance to fatty foods
- Intolerance to alcohol
- Nausea and vomiting attacks
- Abdominal bloating
- Constipation
- Irritable bowel syndrome
- Pain over the liver (upper right corner of abdomen & lower right rib cage)

3. **Blood Sugar Problems**

- Craving for sugar
- Hypoglycaemia and unstable blood sugar levels
- Mature onset diabetes (Type II) is common in those with a fatty liver

4. **Nervous System**

- Depression
- Mood changes such as anger and irritability
- Metaphysically the liver is known as the "seat of anger"
- Poor concentration and "foggy brain"
- Overheating of the body, especially the face and torso

- Recurrent headaches (including migraine) associated with nausea

5. Immune Dysfunction

- Allergies - sinus, hay fever, asthma, dermatitis, hives, etc.
- Multiple food and chemical sensitivities
- Skin rashes and inflammations
- Increased risk of autoimmune diseases
- Chronic Fatigue Syndrome
- Fibromyalgia
- Increase in recurrent viral, bacterial and parasitic infections

6. External Signs

- Coated tongue; bad breath
- Skin rashes; itchy skin (pruritus)
- Excessive sweating; offensive body odour
- Dark circles under the eyes; yellow discolouration of the eyes; red swollen itchy eyes (allergic eyes)
- Acne rosacea (red pimples around the nose, cheeks and chin)
- Brownish spots and blemishes on the skin (liver spots)
- Red palms and soles which may also be itchy and inflamed
- Flushed facial appearance or excessive facial blood vessels (capillaries/ veins)

7. Hormonal Imbalance

- Intolerance to hormone replacement therapy or the contraceptive pill (e.g. side effects)
- Menopausal symptoms such as hot flushes may be more severe
- Premenstrual syndrome may be more severe.

NOTE: All the above symptoms are common manifestations of a dysfunctional liver. However, they can also be due to other causes of a more sinister nature, so in all cases of persistent symptoms it is vital to see your doctor.

Liver Function Tests

There are several liver enzymes that are measured when performing liver function tests, such as:

- **ALT - (alanine aminotransferase)** is an enzyme that is produced in the liver cells (hepatocytes) therefore it is more specific for liver disease than some of the other enzymes. It is generally increased in situations where there is damage to the liver cell membranes. All types of liver inflammation can cause raised ALT. Liver inflammation can be caused by fatty infiltration, some drugs/medications, alcohol, liver and bile duct disease.

- **AST - (aspartate aminotransferase)** which was previously called SGOT. This is a mitochondrial enzyme that is also present in heart, muscle, kidney and brain, therefore it is less specific for liver disease. In many cases of liver inflammation, the AST activity is elevated roughly in a 1:1 ratio.

- **AP - (alkaline phosphatase)** is elevated in many types of liver disease but also in non-liver related diseases. Alkaline phosphatase is an enzyme, or more precisely a family of related enzymes, that is produced in the bile ducts and sinusoidal membranes of the liver but is also present in many other tissues. An elevation in the level of serum alkaline phosphatase is raised in bile duct blockage from any cause. Therefore, raised AP in isolation will generally lead a physician to further investigate this area.

  Conditions such as Primary Biliary Cirrhosis and Sclerosing Cholangitis will generally show a raised AP. Raised levels may also occur in cirrhosis and liver cancer. Alkaline phosphatase is also produced in bone and blood activity.

- **GGT - (gamma glutamyl transpeptidase)** is often elevated in those who use alcohol or other liver toxic substances to excess. An enzyme produced in many tissues as well as the liver. Like alkaline phosphatase, it may be elevated in the serum of patients with bile duct diseases.

Elevations in serum GGT, especially along with elevations in alkaline phosphatase, suggest bile duct disease. Measurement of GGT is an extremely sensitive test, however, and it may be elevated in virtually any liver disease and even sometimes in normal individuals. GGT is also induced by many drugs, including alcohol, therefore often when the AP is normal a raised GGT can often (but not always) indicate alcohol use. Raised GGT can often be seen in cases of fatty liver and also where the patient consumes large amounts of Aspartame (artificial Sweetener) in diet drinks for example.

- **Bilirubin** is the major breakdown product that results from the destruction of old red blood cells (as well as some other sources). It is removed from the blood by the liver, chemically modified by a process call conjugation, secreted into the bile, passed into the intestine and to some extent reabsorbed from the intestine. It is basically the pigment that gives faeces its brown colour.

Bilirubin concentrations are elevated in the blood either by increased production, decreased uptake by the liver, decreased conjugation, decreased secretion from the liver or blockage of the bile ducts.

In cases of increased production, decreased liver uptake or decreased conjugation, the unconjugated or so-called indirect bilirubin will be primarily elevated.

In cases of decreased secretion from the liver or bile duct obstruction, the conjugated or so-called direct bilirubin will be primarily elevated.

Many different liver diseases, as well as conditions other than liver diseases (e.g. increased production by enhanced red blood cell destruction), can cause the serum bilirubin concentration to be elevated. Most adult acquired liver diseases cause impairment in bilirubin secretion from liver cells that cause the direct bilirubin to be elevated in the blood. In chronic, acquired liver diseases, the serum bilirubin concentration is usually normal until a significant amount of liver damage has occurred and cirrhosis is present.

- **Albumin** - Albumin is the major protein that circulates in the bloodstream. As it is made by the liver and secreted into the blood it is a sensitive marker and a valuable guide to the severity of liver disease.

  Low serum albumin concentrations indicate the liver is not synthesizing the protein and is therefore not functioning properly. The serum albumin concentration is usually normal in chronic liver diseases until cirrhosis and significant liver damage is present. There are many other proteins synthesized by the liver however the Albumin is easily, reliably and inexpensively measured.

- **Platelet count** - Platelets are cells that form the primary mechanism in blood clots. They're also the smallest of blood cells. They derived from the bone marrow from the larger cells known as megakaryocytes. Individuals with liver disease develop a large spleen. As this process occurs, platelets are trapped within the sinusoids (small pathways within the spleen). While the trapping of platelets is a normal function for the spleen, in liver disease it becomes exaggerated because of the enlarged spleen (splenomegaly). Subsequently, the platelet count may become diminished.

  Prothrombin time. The prothrombin time is tested to evaluate disorders of blood clotting, usually bleeding. It is a broad screening test for many types of bleeding disorders. When the liver is damaged, it may fail to produce blood clotting factors.

CHAPTER 3:

PHASES OF DETOXIFICATION

There is a lot going on in the body during the detoxification process – most of the work is happening in the largest detoxification organ of the body – the liver. The detoxification phases in the liver are composed of two phases, known as Phase I and Phase II. These phases chemically biotransform toxins into progressively more water-soluble substances through a series of chemical reactions so that they can be excreted from the body.

Phase I: Detoxification
This phase of detoxification usually involves oxidation, reduction, or hydrolysis. A family of enzymes commonly referred to as cytochrome P450 mixed-function oxidases perform the most important processes – detoxifying xenobiotics and endogenous substances.[9]

At least 50 enzymes in 10 families governed by 35 different genes allow Phase I to take place. Many forms of cytochrome P-450 enzymes are involved in Phase I reactions. The highest concentration of cytochrome P-450 occurs in the liver, which is the most active site of metabolism. The lungs and the kidneys are secondary organs of biotransformation, with about one-third of the liver's detoxification capacity. Cytochrome P-450 has also been found in the intestines, adrenal cortex, testes, spleen, heart, muscles, brain, and skin.

---

9 Grant DM. Detoxification pathways of the liver. *J Inher Metab Dis.* 14;421-430, 1991.

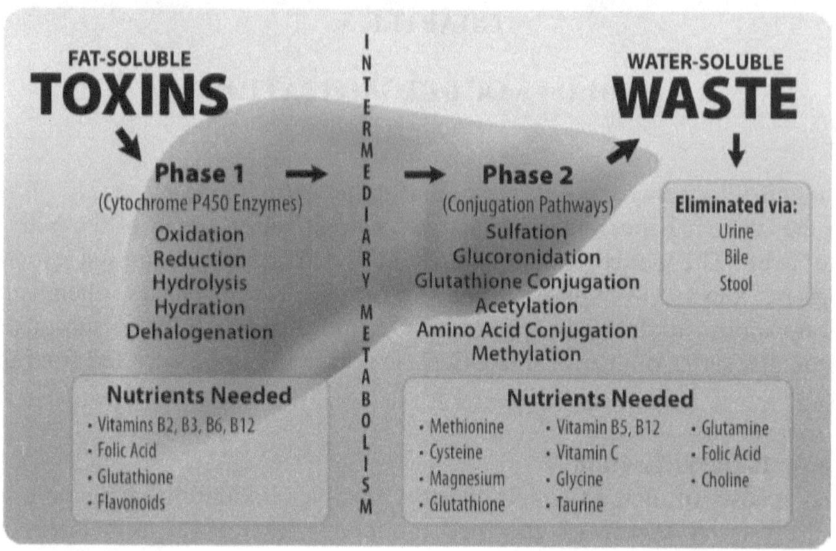

Our understanding of these detoxification pathways over the last couple of decades has helped clinicians understand how they can help patients overcome toxic effects.[10] Sluggish, imbalanced, or impaired detoxification systems can result in the accumulation and deposition of metabolic toxins, increased free radical production and its ensuing pathology, impaired oxidative phosphorylation, and reduced energy.

Nutrients Required for Detoxification Phase
The action of detoxification enzymes in both Phase I and Phase II detoxification pathways depends on the presence of various nutrients.[11,12] For example, alcohol dehydrogenase, an enzyme that converts alcohols (such as ethanol) to aldehydes in an oxidation reaction, depends on an adequate supply of zinc to function properly.

In the next metabolic step, the enzyme aldehyde oxidase changes the aldehyde into an acid that can be excreted in the urine. Aldehyde oxidase depends on an adequate supply of molybdenum and iron. Other minerals

---

10 Davies MH, Gough A, Sorhi RS, Hassel A, Warning R, Emery P. Sulphoxidation and sulphation capacity in patients with primary biliary cirrhosis. *J Hepatol.* 22(5):551-560, May 1995.
11 Anderson KE, Kappas A. Dietary regulation of cytochrome P-450. *Annu Rev Nutr.* 11:141-167, 1991.
12 Bland JS, Bralley JA. Nutritoinal upregulation of hepatic detoxification enzymes. *J Appl Nutr.* 44(3&4):2-15, 1992.

that are required by enzymes include manganese, magnesium, sulfur, selenium, and copper.

Other supporting nutrients involved in cytochrome P-450 enzymes include vitamins B2, B3, B6, B12 and folic acid. The tripeptide glutathione and the branched-chain amino acids leucine, glycine, isoleucine, and valine are also required. Flavonoids and phospholipids are supportive as well.

Protective antioxidant support is required for handling reactive oxygen intermediates produced during Phase I activity. Antioxidant support requires the carotenoids, including beta-carotene, vitamin C and E and coenzyme Q10.

To summarize, the nutrients required during Phase I and Phase II detoxification are:

- ❖ B-complex vitamins: necessary co-factors used in Phase 1 detoxification
- ❖ Digestive enzymes: may be necessary to ensure that protein is adequately digested, and glycine is readily available
- ❖ Essential fatty acids
- ❖ N-acetyl cysteine (NAC): an immediate precursor to glutathione, a potent antioxidant and among the most import detoxification nutrients for the liver
- ❖ Reduced glutathione
- ❖ Selenium, zinc, magnesium and manganese; possibly iron and copper if used with caution
- ❖ Taurine
- ❖ Vitamins C and E and beta carotene
- ❖ Inositol & Methionine: lipotropic agents (help with the breakdown of fat in metabolism) that work to transport fat out of the liver
- ❖ High ORAC vegetable extract blend with polyphenols (a phytonutrient)

Most of these are available in one high-potency multivitamin/mineral formula that we use called HMD MULTIS.[13] The fatty acids can be obtained from KRILL OIL.

In addition, liver herbs can be used to aid detoxification (traditionally known as 'blood cleansing' herbs):

---

[13] www.worldwidehealthcenter.net

❖ Dandelion root, beet leaf & Yellow Dock: cholagogue (stimulates liver secretions and bile flow)
❖ Artichoke leaf: promotes regeneration of the liver and promotes blood flow in that organ; stimulates bile flow
❖ Silymarin (bioflavonoid found in Milk Thistle): according to research, this herbal extract stabilizes the membranes of liver cells, preventing the entry of virus toxins and other toxic compounds including drugs and supports the protection of the liver and promotes its regeneration
❖ Turmeric: a cholagogue like dandelion.
❖ Caraway, dill seeds, sassafras tea

Most of these can be found in the herbal formula that we use called HEPATO PLUS.

Here is a more detailed diagram showing these important nutrients:

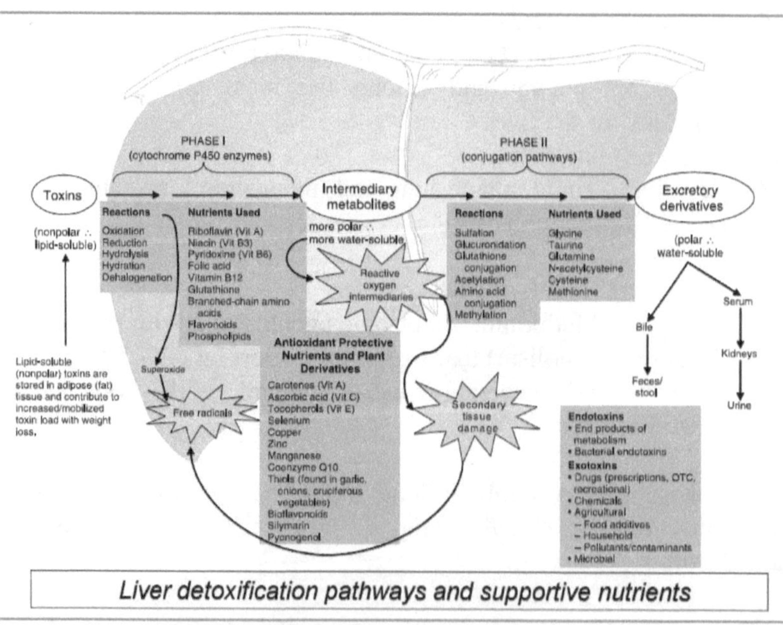

Liver detoxification pathways and supportive nutrients

Usually, the enzymatic reactions in Phase I decrease chemical toxicity. However, toxic or reactive chemicals can form during Phase I that are more toxic than the original compound. This is known as bioactivation. When Phase II detoxification proceeds normally, these chemicals are then rendered harmless and excreted. However, if there is an imbalance in the active levels of Phase I and II detoxifications, these toxins will remain in the body. Imbalance between Phase I and Phase II is associated with increased symptoms of nervous, immune, and endocrine system toxicity.

Toxic chemicals produced during Phase I include teratogens (causing fetus malformation), mutagens (causing cell mutation), and carcinogens (causing cancer). For example, benzo[a]pyrene, a chemical found in coal tar and cigarette smoke, is biologically inert until it is converted by the mixed-function amine oxidase system into a metabolite that can then initiate cancer causing activity. During Phase I, many compounds also form dangerous reactive free radicals - chemicals with an unpaired electron that can cause tissue damage. A buildup of free radicals can increase the risk of cancer.

The level of functioning of Phase I can be measured with a simple caffeine metabolism test. A known quantity of caffeine is ingested, and saliva samples are taken twice at specified intervals. The efficiency of caffeine clearance is directly related to the efficiency of Phase I detoxification. Rapid clearance of caffeine shows enzyme induction (increased production), either from xenobiotic exposure or toxins within the body. A slow rate of caffeine clearance indicates that cytochrome P-450 activity in the liver is abnormal. Patients with slow caffeine clearance have difficulty eliminating xenobiotics and other toxins.

The function of Phase II can be evaluated through the ingestion of both acetaminophen and aspirin. This test measures the recovery of the products of glutathione conjugation, sulfur conjugation, glucuronidation, and glycine conjugation (acylation) in the urine. Comparison to normal values allows evaluation of the efficiency of Phase II. A high ratio between Phase I and any of the Phase II pathways implies imbalanced detoxification in the body.

The detoxification process requires large amounts of caloric energy, which comes mainly from the food we eat. If we do not eat enough protein, the body breaks down vital tissue protein to produce the energy it needs. This decreases the available amounts of Phase I and Phase II enzymes, amino acids, and peptides, because the body breaks down protein to amino acids and peptides. The greater the toxic burden of the body, the higher the need for protein, carbohydrate, fat, and micronutrient intake.

Supplements that Help the Detoxification Pathways
Some of the nutrients required for the proper functioning of the detoxification pathways have already been mentioned above. To reiterate, <u>it is strongly advised that you drink at least 10 glasses of mineral or reverse osmosis water daily</u>, so that you can flush out the toxins quicker.

We have already mentioned taking a multivitamin formula to help optimize your levels of vitamins and minerals, which are crucial raw materials for many of the detoxification pathways of the body. Choose one that has high levels of vitamins and minerals, not just the RDA levels – at the Da Vinci Center we use a high-potency formula called HMD MULTIS.

In addition, taking a couple of grams of vitamin C three times daily during the detoxification process will also help. Vitamin C will help to absorb certain toxins, as well as helping the immune system cope with a heavy burden of toxins that it needs to get rid of. I usually recommend a Calcium/Magnesium Ascorbate in powder form, which is an alkaline form of vitamin C, and is much gentler on the stomach and gut than plain ascorbic acid.

At the Da Vinci Center we use one in capsule form that contains both calcium and magnesium ascorbate, called <u>VITAMIN C BLEND.</u> Take 1 cap x 3 times daily, or you can open these up and place them in some juice or water.

Other supplements that we recommend include the following:
<u>HEPATO PLUS</u> - this is a herbal combination, specifically designed to provide extra support to the detoxification organs and systems of the body – particularly during periods of over-indulgence in food, alcohol or smoking.

Beneficial for...

- Liver cleansing
- A sluggish liver and gallbladder
- Body cleansing and detoxification
- Blood purifying support
- High energy levels
- Cholesterol levels
- Body odour
- Digestive health
- Indigestion
- Relieving symptoms of occasional over-indulgence in food and drink
- A colon cleansing program
- Those with a poor diet
- Those with a high toxic load

You can take one capsule x 3 times daily. Each capsule contains:

- ❖ Artichoke extract (40:1), 2.5% cynarin (equivalent to 4800mg of fresh artichoke)
- ❖ Parsley powder
- ❖ Beetroot extract (5:1) (equivalent to 400mg of fresh beetroot powder)
- ❖ Turmeric powder (95% Curcumin)
- ❖ Burdock root extract (5:1) (equivalent to 200mg of fresh burdock root)
- ❖ Fennel seed extract (4:1) (equivalent to 120mg of fresh fennel seed powder)
- ❖ Dandelion root extract (4:1) (equivalent to 100mg of fresh dandelion root powder)
- ❖ Liquorice root extract (5:1) (equivalent to 100mg of fresh liquorice)
- ❖ N-acetyl L-cysteine
- ❖ Alpha lipoic acid
- ❖ Garlic (black aged garlic) extract (100:1) (equivalent to 500mg of fresh garlic powder)
- ❖ Ginger root powder
- ❖ Cayenne (Capicum Frutescens) extract (8:1) (equivalent to 30mg of fresh cayenne powder)

Another herbal formula called <u>COLFORM</u>. This is a fast-acting, herbal colon cleanser and bowel support formula with 10 active herbal ingredients, including glucomannan.

COLFORM is a well-known herbal colon cleanser and bowel support combination, based on a formula by American master herbalist, Dr. John R. Christopher.

Beneficial for...

- Constipation
- Sluggish bowels
- Haemorrhoids
- Clearing bowel 'pockets'
- Diverticula
- Internal cleansing and detoxification
- Stool softening
- Prior to, following or between colonic hydrotherapy treatments

You should take one capsule x 3 times daily. Each capsule contains:

- ❖ Rhubarb powder
- ❖ Barberry powder
- ❖ Burdock root powder
- ❖ Cayenne powder
- ❖ Ginger root powder
- ❖ Rhubarb root extract (30:1)
- ❖ Fennel seed powder
- ❖ Aloe vera extract (200:1)
- ❖ Clove bud powder
- ❖ Dandelion root extract (4:1)

Another herbal remedy called <u>CONSTFORM</u>, based on one of Dr. John R. Christopher's formulas, is good to add when there has been a history of constipation.

It is a fast-acting colon cleanser, designed for the chronically constipated in need of strong treatment for a blocked bowel.

Beneficial for...

- Chronic constipation
- Internal cleansing
- Lower bowel function
- Bowel regularity
- Laxative abuse
- Use by colonic hydrotherapists before, during and after treatments

You can take one capsule x 3 times daily. Each capsule contains:

- ❖ Rhubarb powder
- ❖ Barberry powder
- ❖ Glucomannan 90%
- ❖ Alfalfa powder
- ❖ Cayenne powder
- ❖ Garlic powder
- ❖ Aloe vera extract (200:1)
- ❖ Dandelion root extract (4:1)
- ❖ Ginger root extract (20:1)

❖   Nettle leaf extract (4:1)

Another herbal formula that I recommend to my patients during the 15-day detox is called <u>PARAFORM PLUS ONE</u>. This one is designed to eliminate parasites from the intestine; we pick these up from food and water all the time, so a couple of times per year it is good to detox from these too.

The ingredients have been hand-picked for their anti-parasitic, anti-bacterial, anti-microbial, anti-fungal and anti-viral activities.

Beneficial for...

- Internal parasites, flukes and worms
- Candida albicans overgrowth
- Irritable Bowel Syndrome (IBS)
- Diarrhoea
- Constipation
- Fungal infections
- Mouth sores and herpes
- Certain skin conditions, such as acne and eczema
- Colon cleansing
- Travel abroad to locations where food hygiene and/or water quality may be less then ideal

Each capsule contains:

❖   Magnesium caprylate – 175mg
❖   Cinnamon powder – 100mg
❖   Cloves powder – 100mg
❖   Shiitake mushroom powder – 100mg
❖   Garlic powder extract (10000mg/g) – 75mg
❖   Glucomannan (95%) – 50mg
❖   Pumpkin seed P E 4:1 (40%) (equivalent to 200 mg pumpkin seed powder) – 50mg
❖   Chicory root P.E 4:1 (equivalent to 120mg chicory root powder) – 30mg
❖   Grapefruit seed P.E 5:1 (equivalent to 100mg grapefruit seed powder) – 20mg
❖   Cayenne extract 7:1 (equivalent to 100mg cayenne powder) – 14.3mg

❖ Fenugreek seed P.E 4:1 (equivalent to 48mg fenugreek seed powder) – 12mg
❖ Olive leaf extract 15:1, 6% Oleurpein (equivalent to 50mg olive leaf powder) – 3.35mg

Yet another supplement that I recommend during the detox that gives the body a good energy boost is called <u>SUPER GREENS PLUS</u>. This is a 100% organic (Soil Association registered) superfoods powder, that can be used as a plant protein powder, light meal shake or daily nutrient booster. In fact, it is one of the most nutrient-dense organic superfood combinations per serving you will find.

It provides a broad range of vitamins, minerals, antioxidants and powerful phyto-nutrients through its multiple organic superfood, superfruit and herbal ingredients.

High in vegetable-source proteins, this full-spectrum blend also contains over 20 natural enzymes and 70 beneficial nutrients.

A great all-round supplement to support energy levels, cleanse, detox, and alkalise the body – daily organic nourishment made easy!
For every 300 g of powder, it contains:

*Activated Pre-Sprouted Barley
*Apple
*Linseed / Flaxseed
*Wheatgrass
*Quinoa
*Barley Grass
*Alfalfa
*Kelp (Ascophyllum)
*Spirulina
*Acai Berry
*Carrot
*Turmeric
*Bilberry Fruit
*Spinach Leaf
*Lemon Peel

Stay with the detoxification process, and allow yourself time to rest, particularly during the first few days. It is best starting on a Friday, given that you will have the weekend at home to get organized and rest when you need to.

I do not recommend vigorous exercise during this initial period, but a 20-30-minute walk with a friend or loved one in an open-air park is fine. You need to conserve your energy levels for the detoxification process. Under normal circumstances, the body uses 80% of its energy for detoxification, which is a substantial amount, and this will increase during the 15 days of this intensive detox programme.

The Good News!
The good news is that after the initial healing crisis you WILL FEEL A LOT BETTER. This is literally a guarantee that I can give you personally, as I have witnessed it hundreds of times with my patients, as well as myself.

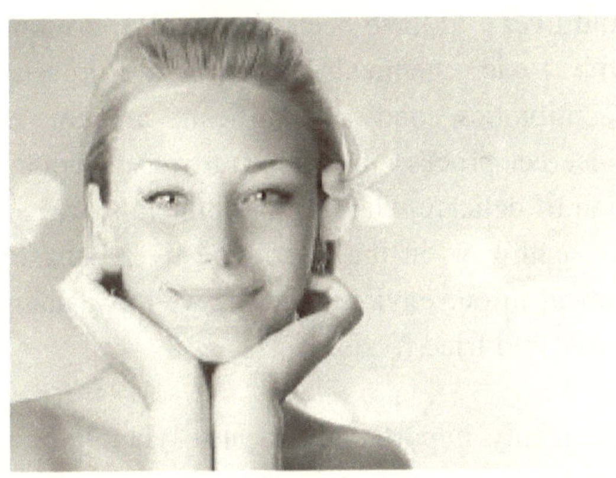

I personally detoxify twice a year for 15 days, and another 7 days in the summer when fruit and juices are plentiful here in Cyprus.

I KNOW how it feels when your body begins to get rid of the toxins and you are over the healing crisis – a clarity of mind that is crystal clear, increased concentration, increased energy levels, better sleep, calmer, more reflective state of being, increased awareness of your environment, better digestion, your constipation improves, body pains dwindle or melt away, arthritis improves, chests and throats clear, skin colour and tone greatly improves and I have had many clients who cut down or actually stopped smoking, as the body rebels harder during a detox programme.

These are all benefits that you will experience, so STICK WITH THE PROGRAMME and achieve OPTIMUM HEALTH. Once you experience this state of optimum health you will wonder what the hell you were doing when you had moderate health, just like most people walking the planet today.

The Alkaline Detox Diet is one of the most positive steps you can take and should be treated and enjoyed that way – treat yourself for 15 days, eat as much as you like, whenever you like, of the foods that you are allowed during the detox.

Liver and Gallbladder Physiology

The liver is the gateway to the body and in this chemical-age its detoxification systems are easily overloaded. Thousands of chemicals are added to food and over 700 have been identified in drinking water. Plants are sprayed with toxic chemicals, animals are injected with potent hormones and antibiotics, and a significant amount of our food is genetically engineered, processed, refined, frozen or cooked. All this can lead to destruction of delicate vitamins and minerals, which are needed for the detoxification pathways in the liver. The liver must try to cope with every toxic chemical in our environment, as well as damaged fats that are present in processed and fried foods.

Therefore it is crucially important to cleanse your liver, much like you clean your house, bedroom, car and external self. Probably cleansing at least once per year is a good thing. When the liver gets overloaded it cannot metabolize fats and cholesterol so easily, and this is when your cholesterol level start increasing and gall stones form, but also the liver itself becomes 'fatty.' Fatty livers are usually found in about 50% of people over the age of 50 – this is often seen by radiologists over time when examining patients routinely. Any imbalances in the liver will have a direct effect on the gallbladder, as it is the liver that produces the bile and gallstones.

Let's look at the gallbladder and how this organ can be easily cleansed, with amazing health benefits.

The gallbladder is a pear-shaped organ that stores about 50 ml of bile until the body needs it for digestion. Bile is a bitter, yellow or green alkaline fluid secreted by hepatoacytes (special cells) in the liver – the human liver can produce close to one litre of bile per day. The bile stored in the gallbladder is between 5-10 times more concentrated and potent that the bile secreted directly by the liver. This bile is discharged into the duodenum (the first part of the small intestine) mainly for the emulsification (breakdown) of fats during digestion – this is why people who have had their gallbladder removed are likely to have a tough time digesting fatty foods.

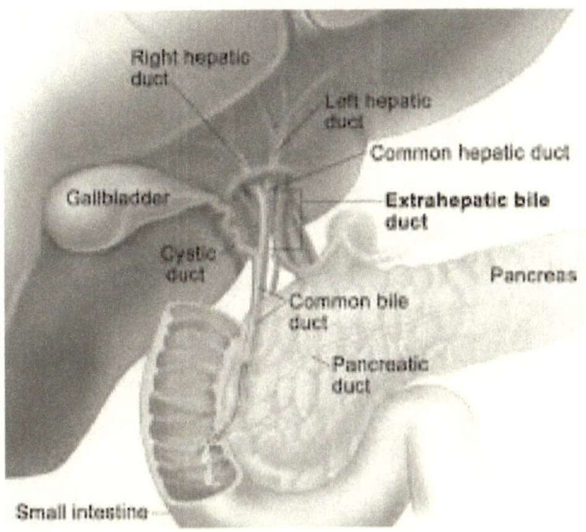

Gallstones

If the tubing of the gallbladder is filled with gallstones, then this can cause several health problems including allergies or hives. However, some people have no symptoms. These stones cannot be seen by ultrasound scan or X-rays as they are not actually in the gallbladder, but in the ducts. They may also not be calcified stones. There are many types of gallstones, most of which have cholesterol crystals in them. They can be black, red, white, green or tan coloured.

As the stones grow and become more numerous, the back-pressure on the liver causes it to make less bile. This is also thought to slow the flow of lymphatic fluid. Imagine if your garden hose had small stones in it; the result would be that much less water would flow. When there are gallstones present, much less cholesterol leaves the body, resulting in elevated cholesterol levels.

Moreover, gallstones are porous so can pick up all the bacteria, cysts, viruses and parasites that are passing through the liver. These masses or 'nests' of infectious material hang around the liver and supply the blood flowing through it with lots of fresh bugs daily. This is one way that parasites are circulated and reproduce. These parasites and infectious nests must be removed, and the simplest way of doing that is to remove the gallstones.

There are several levels of detoxification that will be discussed – at the Da Vinci Center I recommend that my patients go through these detoxification regimes, before jumping directly into the gallbladder cleanse. In fact, it is rare that a patient walks into my office and begins the gallbladder cleanse from the first day.

Usually, these are the detox protocols that I suggest in chronological order:

1. All-body 15-day Da Vinci Alkaline detoxification diet
2. Parasite detox
3. Heavy metal detox
4. Gallbladder and liver cleanse
5. Other detox regimes as required (each patient differs).

So, let us begin by looking at some of the preparations that we need to make in order to be ready and fully understand what we will be doing, and why.

Before Starting the Detox Programme
There are a few indications which would exclude some people from starting the detox programme and you should not do so if any of the following apply:

❖ You are pregnant – the toxins released during the detoxification process can harm the embryo because the embryo's capacity to detoxify is limited due to its poor organ functionality at such early stages of development.

❖ You are breastfeeding – toxins released into the mother's blood will travel to the milk, so the baby will get a dose of toxic milk that will not help them in any way. Wait until after the baby is weaned off the breast and meanwhile you could start eating healthily.

❖ You are presently being treated for an illness or condition such as diabetes or heart problems without medical supervision. It is important for your doctor or health practitioner to know what you are doing. With diabetics, for example, it is possible that you might go into a hypoglycemic episode where your blood sugar levels fall below normal, due to the increased insulin production by the pancreas.

I have seen this several times – as the pancreas begins to clear of toxic overloads, it begins to function better, so it can begin to produce MORE insulin than before, resulting in a sudden decrease of blood sugar levels. This is fine if a health practitioner is aware of what is going on, and can adjust the dosage of drugs to suit.

❖ You are recovering from a serious illness without expert medical supervision – if you are recovering from cancer, any type of operation, an accident or other serious disease, then you should be extremely careful of detoxifying by yourself. The toxins released in the body could upset the healing process and period of convalescence. Seek guidance from an experienced health practitioner who has experience in detoxifying. It is pointless asking a doctor who has no idea of detoxifying, as you are more than likely going to get a negative report, just from pure ignorance. Seek the help of an experienced person in these matters and take note that not many medical doctors are knowledgeable of the detoxification process, nor have experience in these matters. Only very few do, so do not take it for granted that all are knowledgeable because they are doctors.

❖ You are taking any prescribed or non-prescribed medication – again, the toxins mixed with the drugs could exacerbate further the healing crisis and cause more symptoms than are necessary.

❖ You are not ready at this moment in time to begin – the detox programme does require a little discipline and organization so would not be suited to a person who is travelling continuously, or eating out continuously with business associates, or who is under a lot of stress from marital or domestic problems. We need to prepare ourselves psychologically and emotionally before we begin. If you feel that this is not the right time for you, then postpone it for another time when you are ready.

CHAPTER 4:

PREPARING FOR DETOX

Preparing for the detox is not difficult, nor is it costly, but should be done some time BEFORE you decide to begin. There are several things that you need to gather before you start. A checklist of essentials is outlined below:

- ❖ A large stock of fresh vegetables and fruit in season – kept in the fridge for freshness. If you have access to ORGANIC FRUIT and VEGETABLES, then this should be your obvious first choice. Organic produce is free from the pesticides and chemical fertilizers that are harmful to the body but are also richer in nutrients due to the organic fertilizers that are used. One famous doctor, Dr. Gerson, said, *"The soil is our second metabolism."* What he meant by this profound statement was that the nutrient quantity and quality of the soil is going to determine the quality of our bodily functioning. Organic produce has been 'fed' the right ingredients of minerals, trace elements and vitamins that our bodies require to function optimally.

I sincerely wish I had a steady supply of organic produce at my disposal here in Cyprus where I work and live, but unfortunately, we are not that health conscious as a nation to begin organic farming yet.

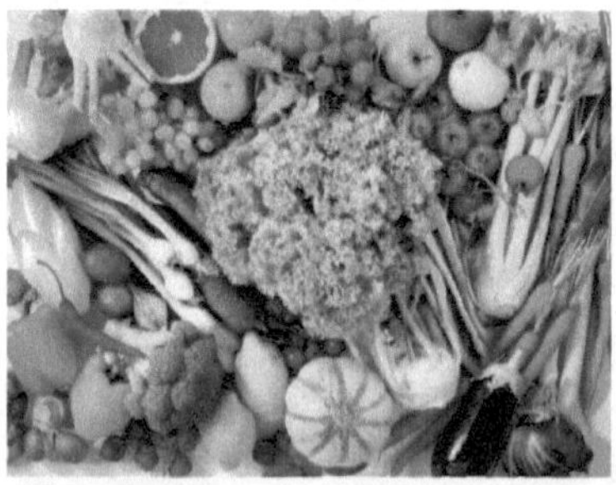

- ❖ A good thermos flask – you can use this for transporting freshly squeezed fruit or vegetable juices to and from work. It is important to remember, however, that the live enzymes and vital energy in freshly squeezed juices have a life-span of ONLY THREE HOURS. So, it is crucial that you drink the juice within these 3 hours and try to keep the juice as cool as possible – heat can destroy these very vulnerable enzymes. You may also use the flask to transport herbal teas, either hot or cold (with ice cubes) if you wish.

❖ A good quality juicer – there are many different types of juicers on the market, and it is a true science to choose the right one. Most of the juicers on the market for domestic use are centrifugal juicers. If you are buying one, try to find the best that money will buy as this is going to be a sound health investment that will see you through many years of life. There are cheaper ones at half the price that will probably only last a year or less, so choose carefully. You could pick up a good one for less than $100, but if you can pay to buy the Rolls Royce of juicers, go for something like a Champion juicer (about $300), which will extract 25% more nutrients from vegetables and juices than the centrifugal juicer. The Champion juicer is a masticating juicer – it grinds the fruit or vegetable into a paste before spinning at high speed, to squeeze the juice through a screen set into the juicer bottom. The ultimate in juicers is the Health Stream Press which can extract up to 50% more juice than a centrifugal juicer but can cost from $500 to over $2,000 for the automated press.

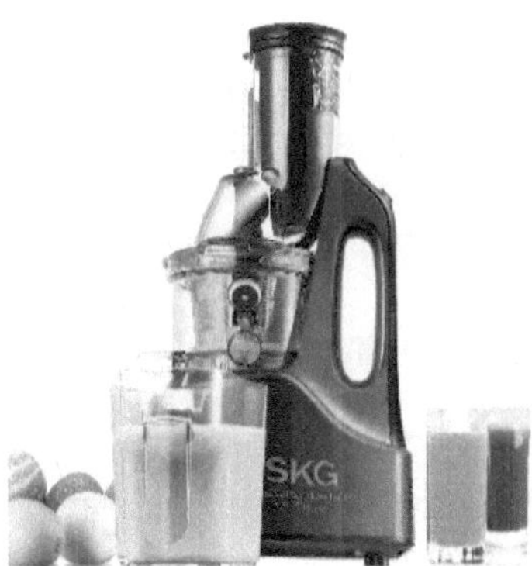

❖ A steamer – metal (stainless steel) or bamboo – the type you place over or in the pan of hot water to steam vegetables. Steaming is far more preferable to boiling because when you boil vegetables in water, they lose minerals such as potassium, which is crucial to health. Steaming vegetables decreases the losses of these important minerals.

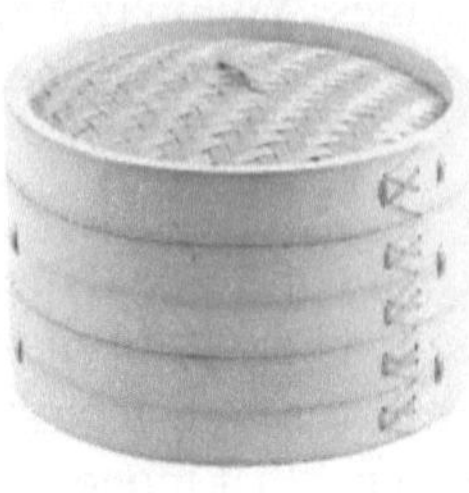 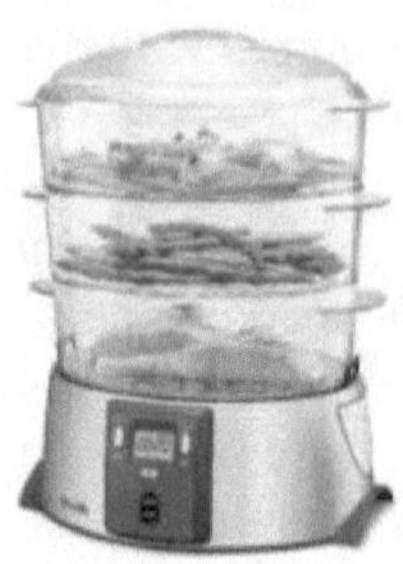

❖ Extra virgin olive oil – this is extracted using a cold press method from whole, ripe, undamaged olives. It is made without heat and is unrefined, as compared with olive oil that is not virgin or extra virgin. It still contains many of the natural factors unique to olives, which are normally lost through degumming, refining, bleaching and deodorizing. Virgin olive oils do not suffer nutrient losses and molecular changes that negatively affect human health. Choose this oil over ones that do not have the word 'virgin' or 'extra virgin' on the label.

❖ Fresh garlic – have plenty of fresh garlic at hand - it would be wise to eat one clove a day as this contains more than 200 chemical compounds, most of them having therapeutic qualities. Eating fresh parsley and lemon juice or sucking on a whole clove can help to neutralize garlic odour on the breath. Garlic can inhibit and kill bacteria, fungi and parasites; lower blood pressure, blood cholesterol and blood sugar; prevent blood clotting; protect the liver and contains anti-tumour properties. It can also boost the immune system to fight off potential disease and maintain health.

Regarding detoxification, which particularly interests us here, garlic can stimulate the lymphatic system, which expedites the removal of waste from the body. It can nourish most of the organs such as the heart, stomach, circulation and lungs, as well as protect the cells from damage by nasty free radicals (molecules that harm the body). The sulphur elements in garlic also help to stimulate certain enzyme systems that are beneficial for detoxifying, such as the liver's glutathione pathways, which help to remove toxins from the body; there are going to be plenty of these passing through the liver in the next 15 days.

So, now you understand why garlic is so important. It is one of the true wonders of nature, and I cannot understand why people dismiss it because of its odour, yet we accept so many other disgusting smells such as smokers smelling like ashtrays!

❖ A brush made of natural fibre – this is going to be used for SKIN BRUSHING (see details below).

❖ Water – you will need a large supply of either mineral or distilled water throughout the detoxification process. I suggest that you drink at least 10 glasses daily – this may mean having a glass next to you at home and the workplace and keeping it topped up. You will be surprised how many glasses you can drink in a day if you do this systematically. It really is a matter of habit, but what I have found is that if you don't have the water to hand, you will not remember to drink it. Water is crucial to detoxification. It is part of the flushing process, which gets the toxins that are released by the cells out of the body. After a lot of research regarding water filters, I have personally settled for the reverse osmosis unit with a vortex energizer – there are many companies now that can fit the unit under your sink and add a separate small tap specifically for the drinking water. This is connected to your tap water, but the reverse osmosis filter will eliminate literally everything from chlorine, fluoride, heavy metals, pesticide residues as well as micro-organisms – it is squeaky clean water that you can drink and cook with.

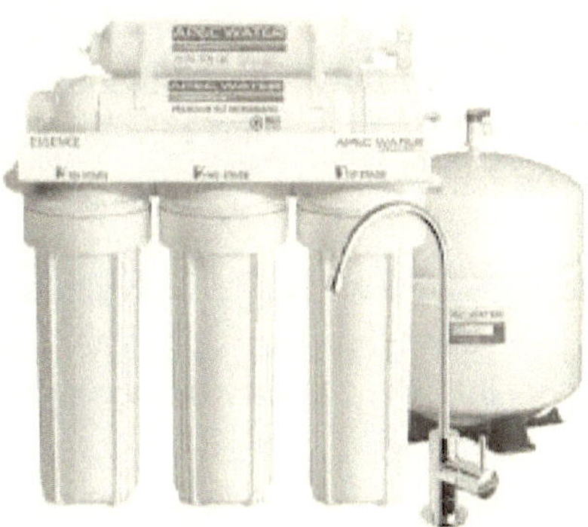

❖ Fresh lemons or cider vinegar – what you use is really a matter of taste, but both are excellent and healthy condiments. Cider vinegar made from apples is very rich in potassium, a mineral that is required by all cells during metabolism. In his book, *'Cider Vinegar'*, Cyril Scott talks about how cider vinegar can help overweight people, citing several case histories. He recommends two teaspoons of cider vinegar in a tumbler of water, to be taken on rising in the morning. Exactly how it works is an enigma, but even if it does not work for weight loss, it will certainly help to alkalize the blood and help clean it.

❖ Herbal teas – there are several herbal teas that you could drink every day throughout the detox programme. Green tea is excellent. Apart from being rich in vitamin A, E, C, calcium and iron, it contains healthy phytonutrients called Epigallocatechin Gallate (EGCG), which inhibit the growth of cancer and lowers cholesterol levels. Dandelion 'coffee' is also excellent, as this herb purifies the blood, detoxifies and stimulates the function of the liver. It's also a natural diuretic. It's good to drink teas that help to drain the detoxification organs and get rid of the toxins. Another good one is stinging nettle tea, which helps to drive excess fluid out of the tissues and helps with metabolism by increasing the elimination through the kidneys. Other goodies are chamomile, peppermint, rosehip, blackcurrant, elder flower, strawberry and Melissa. Most of these can be found in good health food shops – either in tea bags, or loose.

Major detoxification centres of the body

The toxins will be released through four major detoxification centres of the body – the more you can help these detoxification pathways to open, the less detox symptoms you will have. The major detoxification organs/centres of the body are:

1. **Skin** – excretes toxins such as DDT, heavy metals and lead through sweat. Skin brushing and saunas, as well as infrared saunas, are good ways of opening the skin pores in order for toxins to be released.

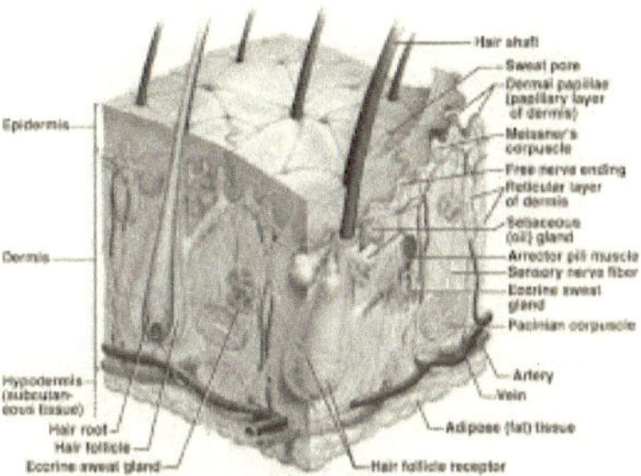

2. Liver – filters the blood to rid it of bacteria; secretes bile to rid the blood of cholesterol, haemoglobin breakdown products and excess calcium. It also gets rid of prescription drugs from amphetamines, digitalis, nicotine, sulphonamides, acetaminophens, morphine and diazepam. There are good herbs that can open up the detox channels in the liver such as dandelion (Taraxacum officinale), milk thistle (Silybum marianum), Green tea (Camellia sinensis), Artichoke (Cynara scolymus), Methionine, N-Acetyl Cysteine and Alpha lipoic acid and others.

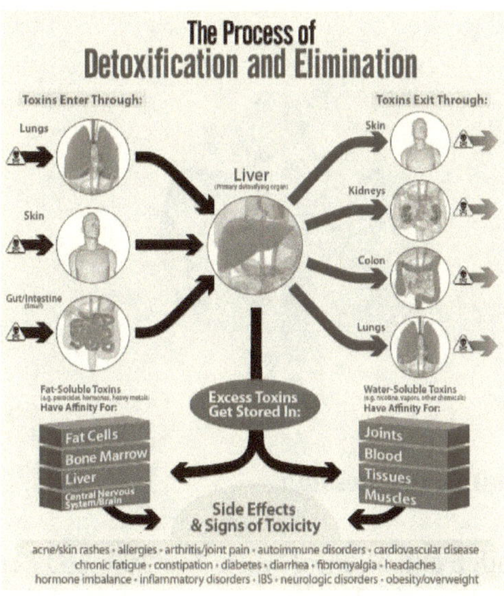

3. Intestine – mucosal detoxification to rid toxins from bowel bacteria; and excretion through faeces of fat-soluble toxins excreted in the bile.

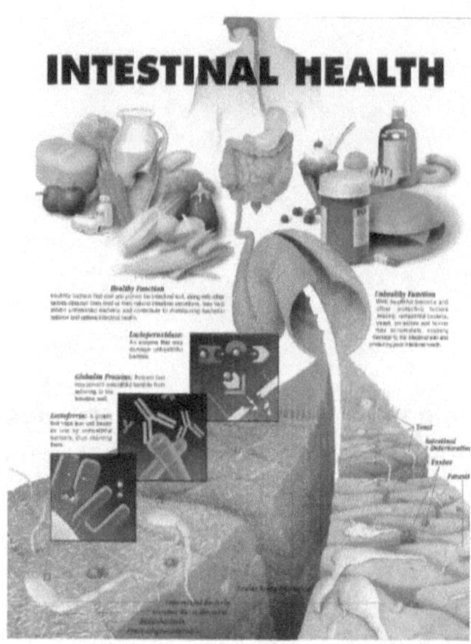

4. **Kidneys** – excretion through urine of toxins after they are made water-soluble by the liver.

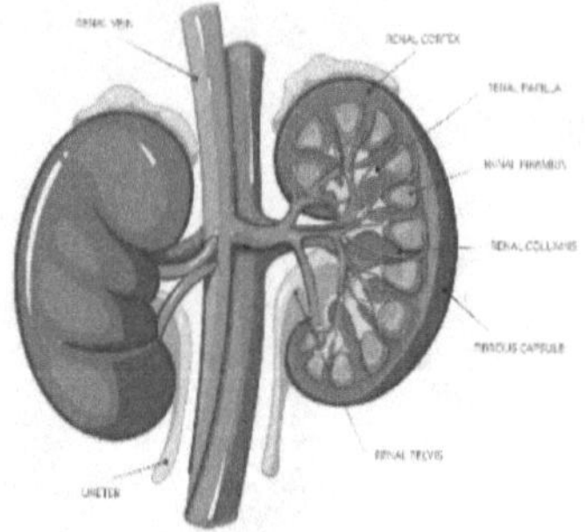

Food Enzymes and Detoxification

To remove the sludge and harmful waste from the body cells and tissues, it is important that you eat foods rich in live enzymes such as fresh fruits and vegetables and their fresh juices. These are dynamic catalytic substances that have the power to break down the fatty wastes stubbornly clinging to your fat cells and wash them out of the body. Food enzymes scrub your cells clean and therefore slim them down, and consequently slimming you down too.

Thorough chewing is a unique way of detoxifying the sludge from the mucous membranes of the gastrointestinal tract (GI). Whenever we chew, an enzyme called *urogastrone* is released which can help digest sludge present on the mucous membranes as well as offering a protective coating of the GI to protect against erosion.

Initially, science thought of enzymes as dead chemicals that merely acted as catalysts – making things work faster. Since then, the works of people like Dr. Edward Howell: 'Enzyme nutrition' and Anthony Cichoke: 'Enzymes and enzyme therapy,' has shown that enzymes are indeed very much alive and have lots of stored potential energy. As Dr. Howell states in his book, 'They are protein carriers charged with vital energy factors, just as your car battery consists of metal plates charged with electrical energy.'

These enzymes help you to digest your food, to absorb nutrients into your bloodstream and to dispatch nutrients to every part of your body. Without enzymes, there would be no life! These live enzymes with this vital energy come only from raw, live foods or their juices. Since good health depends on all metabolic enzymes doing an excellent job, we must make sure that nothing interferes with the body making enough of them.

One of the problems with maintaining the level of these enzymes is that they are very sensitive to heat – they are intolerant of heat. If water is hot enough to feel uncomfortable to the hand, it will injure enzymes in food. Nearly all the food that we eat is cooked – most of it is cooked to death! Cooked food is deficient in enzymes with their vital energy. This means that you are also deficient in enzymes, which will lead to incompletely metabolized food (which is stored as waste in your adipocytes), giving you excess weight.

It is therefore crucially important to attack the stored-up sludge in your adipose tissue mass. So how do we get a good source of live enzymes? – we eat live, raw foods.

If there are digestive problems such as bowel distension, bloating, flatulence and wind, pain after eating – it would be wise to supplement a digestive enzyme with your food – we use one called DIGEST PLUS. You will find that as the food is digested your bloating will be a thing of the past in 15-20 days but carry on taking the digestive enzymes for at least 3 months.

If there are also a difficulty digesting protein concentrates such as meat and pulses, then this is an indication of hypochlorhydria or an insufficient production of hydrochloric acid by the stomach. This will cause stomach bloating, a feeling of heaviness after eating protein foods that will last many hours. This is because the stomach must keep the food there for many hours to digest it correctly and you are likely to get fermentation, and wind will be expelled by mouth. In this case, you will also need to take Betaine hydrochloric acid and Pepsin capsules with food – we use the formulation called BETAINE COMPLEX.

Before embarking on the gallbladder cleanse, it would be good to go through a more thorough all-body cleanse as discussed below, as well as the parasite and heavy metal detox – all these can run in parallel to really clean many of the toxins that have probably resulted in the gallbladder stones.

Let's look at the Da Vinci Alkaline Detoxification Diet that I have personally supervised tens of thousands of patients to go through throughout the years. Indeed, I often recommend to my patients to repeat this procedure every 6 months in order to keep the toxins at bay.

65

CHAPTER 5:

THE DA VINCI CENTRE DETOXIFICATION DIET
CLEAN, CLEAN, CLEAN!

The 15-day Alkaline Detoxification Diet (15-DADD)

Most of the patients that come to me for a wide variety of health problems will be placed on the Da Vinci Centre's 15-day Alkaline Detoxification Diet (15-DADD). This is a diet that I have put together through clinical experience, as well as studying the work of other practitioners[14,15,16,17] who are very well versed in the field of detoxification.

Most of my patients can safely follow this 15-day detoxification programme, except for a few who have other diseases such as diabetes, cancer, heart conditions, low blood pressure and some neurological diseases. There are modified protocols for all the aforementioned, but these should be supervised by a qualified health practitioner.

These more complex patients need more thought and each detoxification regime can be tailored to suit each patient. Therefore, I take a careful history from each one, as well as examining all their clinical findings. These include blood tests, blood pressure, conducting an Iridology examination (looking at the iris, the coloured part of the eye, using an iris microscope which gives me further health information), as well as other diagnostic instruments that I have at my disposal such as Live Blood Analysis, VEGA testing, Biological Terrain Analysis, heavy metal testing, Autonomic Response Testing, Thermography and more[18].

---

[14] Ballie-Hamilton, P. The Detox diet. UK: Penguin, 2002.

[15] Scrivner, J. Detox Yourself. UK: Judy Piatkus (Publishers) Ltd., 1998.

[16] Wade, C. Inner Cleansing: How to Free Yourself from the Joint-Muscle-Artery-Circulation Sludge. New York: Parker Publishing Co., 1992.

[17] Cabot, S. Juice Fasting Detoxification. USA: The Sprout House, 1992.

[18] www.naturaltherapycenter.com

Generally, most patients will be able to tell me what their problem is and its severity, as they have usually received a medical diagnosis before arriving on my doorstep.

Given that all is OK to begin the 15-day detox diet, I suggest that they eat only fresh fruit, salads, freshly squeezed juices, steamed vegetables and vegetable soups for 15 consecutive days. This means that they ONLY eat these foods for the duration, most of which will be rich in the live enzymes, which are the tools required to flush out the toxins from the body. You must be patient and put your mind to it.

I cannot emphasize just how important the detoxification diet is to your success!

What will I be eating during the 15-DADD?
I strongly suggest that you try to eat as many raw fruits and vegetables as possible, including at least 1-3 fruit and vegetable juices daily. Carrot juice has a strong effect on the digestive system, provides energy, serves as an important source of minerals, promotes normal elimination, has diuretic properties and helps to build healthy tissue, skin and teeth. So,

I recommend as many carrot juices as they can handle, mixed with beetroot juice (about 1/3rd of a glass), which are powerful cleansing agents of the body. Beets are said to really cleanse the blood and kidneys. In nature, homogenous colours do not occur by accident – it is no coincidence that the red beetroot affects the blood!

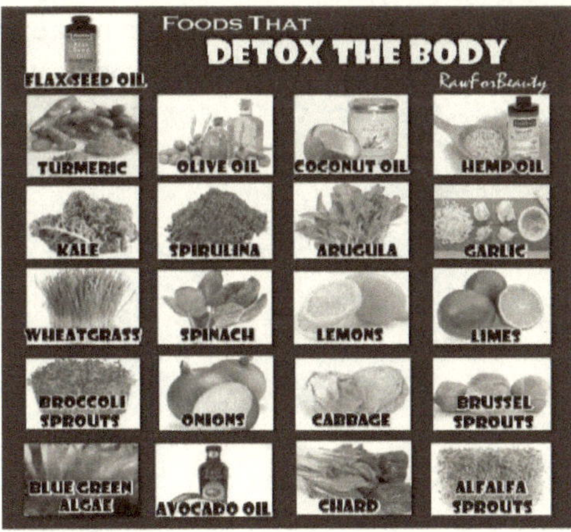

I also encourage the use of a little 'green juice' mixed with each carrot juice. This can be anything from fresh parsley, lettuce, kale, collard greens, Swiss chard, alfalfa, cabbage, spinach, turnip greens, watercress, celery, cucumber, green pepper, scallions, coriander, or any other green vegetable in season. You can place a couple of inches of the green juice in the glass, and top up with carrot juice. All green vegetables contain chlorophyll, which is very oxygenating for the body. It is also an effective antiseptic, cell stimulator, red blood builder and rejuvenator – therefore helping to remove toxic sludge faster. Greens are also super-rich in live enzymes.

I also suggest that each meal should begin with raw fruit or vegetables, seasoned with a little lemon, ginger, garlic, coconut or desired herbs. This way, they are available for digesting the fat, protein, and carbohydrates from the meal that follows. The enzymes in vegetables control or restrict the amount of waste deposited on your adipocytes. Remember to chew all foods thoroughly.

These are the foods that I allow during the detoxification phase – no other family of foods is allowed. You may eat as many of the following foods as you wish, but it is best to eat only when you feel hungry. Wash all fruit and vegetables in a bowl of water with 4-5 tablespoons of grape vinegar added (not apple cider vinegar), to help wash away any pesticide/herbicide residues. Rinse afterwards with clean water. Here are the foods that you can eat in plenty – in fact, the more you eat and drink, the quicker you detoxify:

• **SALADS** – use any type of fresh vegetables you like, in any combination. Use organic vegetables when available and include bean sprouts when in season. Salad dressings should be kept simple – a little virgin olive oil with fresh lemon or lime juice, or cider vinegar. Add plenty of fresh onion and garlic – these are very detoxifying!

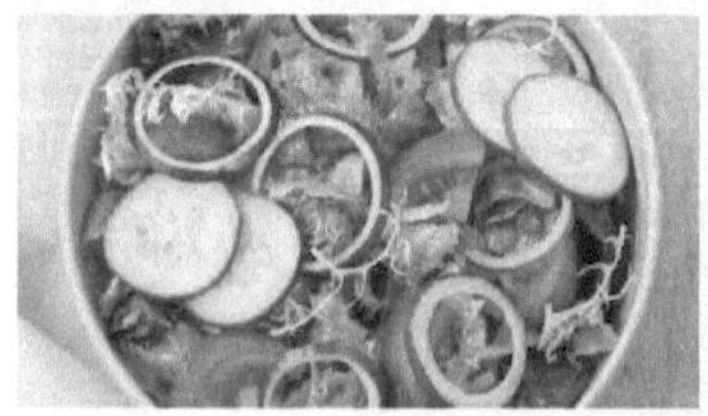

• **STEAMED VEGETABLES** – eat any variety you like, including broccoli, cauliflower, potatoes, beetroot, carrots, etc. Steam as opposed to boil, and eat with a little herbal salt, lemon and a little virgin olive oil, with plenty of garlic. You may also have jacket potatoes with a little olive oil, garlic and parsley dressing.

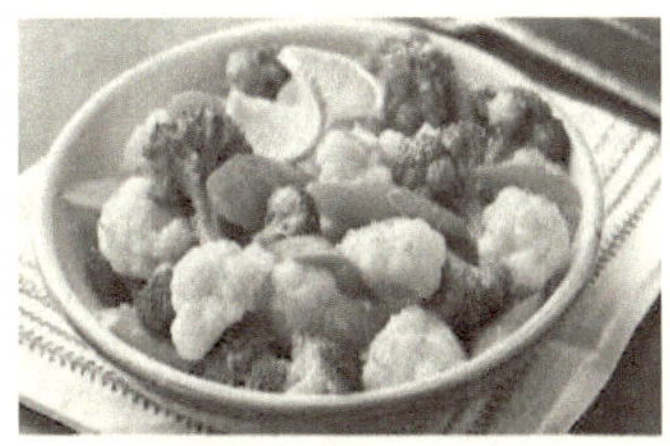

• **STIR-FRIED VEGETABLES** – this is a quick, easy way of cooking vegetables healthily. Use no more than four cups of chopped, hard or medium-hard vegetables or eight to twelve cups chopped leafy greens in a 14-inch wok to avoid crowding the pan. It's important that the vegetables are very dry, otherwise, the vegetables will steam and braise in the pan and lose their crisp texture. Giving the vegetables a whirl in a salad spinner is the easiest solution, but you can also pat them thoroughly with kitchen towels.

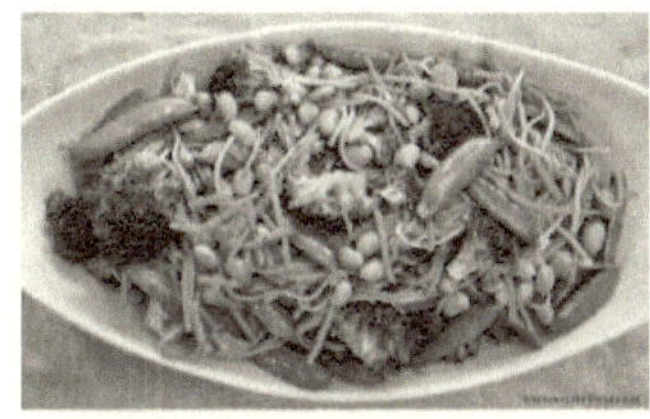

• **VEGETABLE SOUPS** – again quick and easy to make, and very nutritious, providing all the vegetables that our bodies require. It is easy to digest and is generally low in calories. Studies have shown that we tend to eat 20% less calories overall when we eat soups before a main meal. You can make nutritious leak and broccoli soups, as well as tomato and clear soups with various vegetables, adding onion and garlic for their detoxification benefits too.

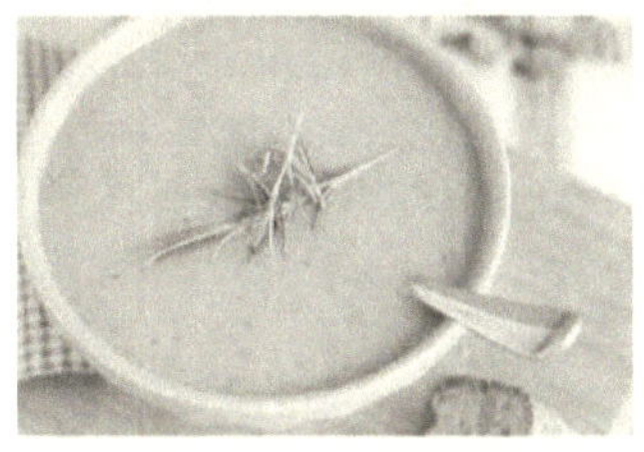

• **VEGETABLE/FRUIT JUICES** – drink a minimum of 1-3 per day and try to include one cocktail comprising one-third of a glass of raw, green juice (spinach, parsley, cabbage and any other green vegetables), topped up with carrot juice. There is no limit to the amount of fresh vegetable and fruit juices that you may drink in a day.

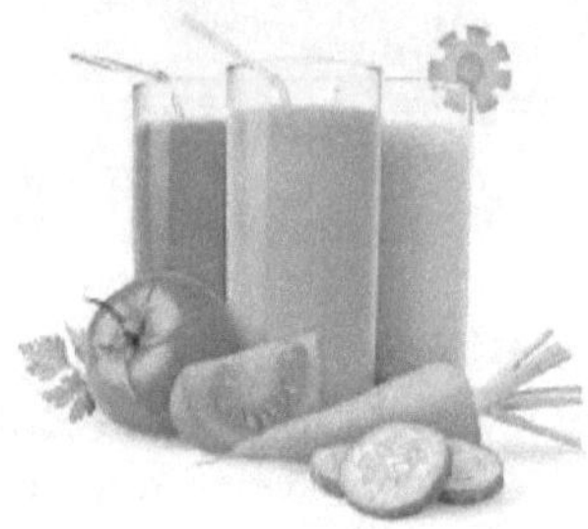

• **FRESH FRUIT** – choose the fruit of your choice (preferably organic) and eat as much as you like, whenever you like. You could begin the day with 2-3 pieces of fruit, which are gentle on the digestive system. Make a tasty fruit salad and eat it in the morning as this helps to detoxify. Fruit is rich in antioxidant phytonutrients which are beneficial to the body in many ways; protecting us from chronic diseases.

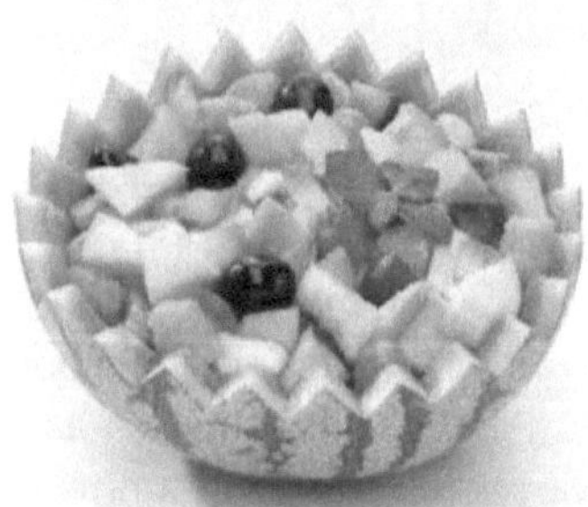

• **HERBAL TEAS** – choose any of your choice. Chamomile is a good relaxant; aniseed and mint is good for the digestive system; Kombucha; dandelion tea or 'coffee' (which is excellent for purifying the blood and detoxifying and stimulating liver function); Sage tea, (which is a blood cleanser); or Nettle tea, (which is excellent for driving away excess fluid out of the tissues and is a wonderful cleanser for all the detoxification organs). Drink as many as you like, with a little honey on the tip of a teaspoon if you like, but plain is best.

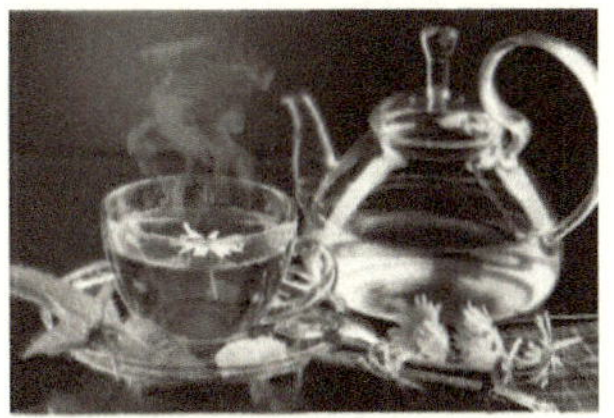

You will also need to drink at least 8-10 glasses per day of still mineral water to flush out the toxins – this is VERY IMPORTANT, so please take note!

When the 15 days are over, you should carry on eating the above for a couple more days while gently adding a little protein such as fresh steamed or grilled fish, organic chicken, pulses, a soft-boiled organic egg or a little cheese. Go gently on the protein for a couple of days before you begin eating normally again so that you do not overload your digestive system.

Lots of Food and Calories

This may appear to be an awful lot of calories, since there are no restrictions on the amount of such foods consumed over the 15-day period. The purpose of this diet, however, is to DETOXIFY – to remove the toxins from the fat cells and tissues as well as the organs, so that the body can return to its optimum level of functionality. I have yet to see anyone going through the 15-DADD put on any weight, so don't worry about counting calories – most people lose one or more kilos (2-4 lbs) over the 15-day period.

I had one gentleman weighing 150 kg (nearly 24 stone) who lost 10 kg (22 lbs) in 15 days, but I believe that most of this was accumulated fluid due to a drinking problem. On a biochemical and microbiological level, there is much going on during the detoxification.

The pH or acidity/alkalinity of the body is being adjusted back to normal, and any nasty pathogens in the body are encouraged to reverse their course. This is based on the work of Enderlein, Neissens and Beauchamp who were proponents of pleomorphism as opposed to monomorphism.

With our bad eating, smoking and drinking habits, body chemistry is unbalanced in most people. This unbalanced body chemistry will be another metabolism blocker that will not allow the body to digest, assimilate, eliminate or get rid of fatty deposits optimally.

Detoxification Symptoms: "The healing crisis"
When the body detoxifies, it goes through various biochemical and physiological changes.[19] Generally, on the first day of fasting the blood sugar level is likely to drop below 65-70 mg/dl. The liver immediately compensates by converting glycogen to glucose and releasing it in the blood. After a few hours, the basal metabolic rate is likely to fall to conserve energy. This means that the heart, pulse and blood pressure will drop. More glycogen may be used from muscles, causing some weakness.

Most common detox symptoms:	
• Sweating	• Restlessness
• Diarrhoea	• Hot and cold flushes
• Vomiting	• Stomach cramps
• Nausea	• Disturbed, or no sleep
• Delirium	• Inability to get warm
• Irritability	• Intense cravings

As the body requires more energy, some fat and fatty acids are broken down to release glycerol from the glyceride molecules and are converted to glucose. You may notice the skin becoming quite oily as these fatty acids and glycerol increase in the blood. The skin is one of the largest detoxification organs, so you may get some skin problems such as pimples, acnes or a pussy boil – this is all part of the body trying to cleanse. The complexion may become pallid for a day or two as the wastes accumulate in the blood.

The incomplete oxidation of fats may result in the formation of Ketones resulting in ketoacidosis. Combined with high levels of urea, resulting from protein metabolism, this state can cause several symptoms which may suppress appetite; they affect the satiety centre in the hypothalamus.

Generally, this takes a few days to happen and you may notice your appetite dwindling. You may get pains in different joints, or organs such as the lungs. There may be a considerable amount of yellow mucus released

---

19 Salloum, TK. Fasting Signs and Symptoms: A Clinical Guide. USA: Buckeye Naturopathic Press, 1992.

from the throat and expelled. The sinuses may also begin clearing with more mucus secreted.

Given that the body is releasing these toxins quickly during the first few days of the detoxification process, it should not surprise you to experience some changes in your body that may cause certain symptoms. Initially, for the first 2-3 days these symptoms can be a little unpleasant, SO BE WARNED!

A fair number of people will have headaches, nervousness, diarrhoea, upset stomach, energy loss, furry tongue, halitosis (bad breath), as well as acne or other skin rashes, a general feeling of malaise, frequent urination due to the toxins irritating the bladder and some of their existing symptoms may be exacerbated. When the toxic residues enter the blood, they affect mind and body functions.

These may be unpleasant symptoms for the first couple of days, but they are a NORMAL part of the detoxification process, and in natural medicine we call this the HEALING CRISIS. All these symptoms indicate that the DETOX IS WORKING! This is a temporary and transient crisis, it will pass – so hang on in there and don't worry that there is something wrong with you.

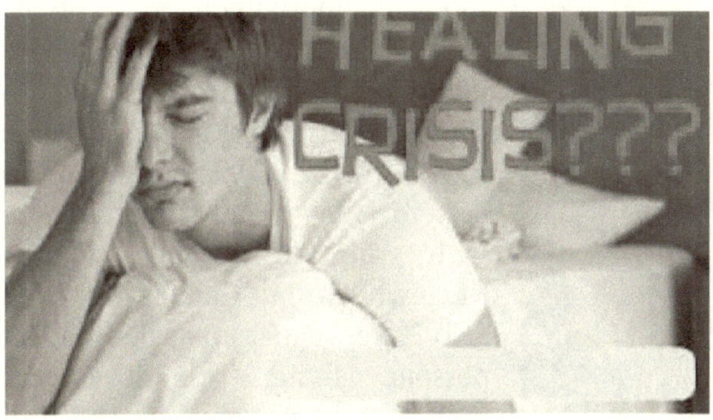

There was always something wrong with you, and now you are doing something about it – you are reversing this toxic process that your body has adapted to.

If you are a coffee drinker, then the symptoms will be more pronounced, as your body will be in a state of withdrawal. Yes, coffee is a drug and when you come off it you go into withdrawal, meaning that your body will start asking for a dose of what it is addicted to. When it doesn't get it, then it screams for it louder and louder, usually in the form of headaches, migraines, muscle pains, general weakness and lack of concentration.

Enduring a cleansing crisis is the hardest part of the healing process. To stop feeling bad, most people want to eat, but do not eat during a cleansing crisis! The body is overloaded with the work of removing toxins. Digestion makes matters worse. Drinking one or two glasses of sodium bicarbonate (baking soda) – one teaspoon in each glass drunk twice daily - will help to neutralize the ketoacidosis.

Helter-skelter rides are common – the 'downward slope' is when the body is vigorously cleansing, and the blood gets swamped with toxins causing you to feel down, moody, depressed and achy, like having a bad cold. You feel weak and lethargic. The mind rationalizes: 'I feel horrible: this can't be working.' You can maintain a normal routine of work on a dip but it requires willpower and determination. It also helps to know that the longer the down period, the greater the fasting high

Killing Uninvited Guests: The Parasite Cleanse!

A perfect combination with the 15-day alkaline detoxification diet is to take some herbs to help eliminate parasites that we are accumulating from our food and environment on a daily basis.

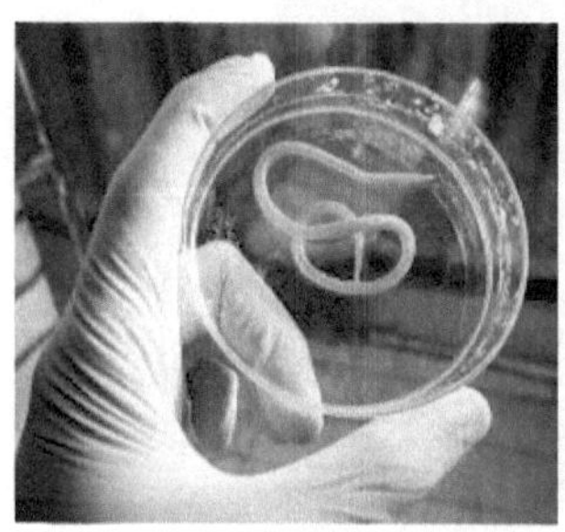

Schmidt and Roberts in their 1989 'Foundations of parasitology'[20] book noted that 25% – 30% of people living in the south-eastern US – mainly children – were infected with whip worm (the trichuris species)[21]. Meanwhile, the Centers of Disease Control also stress that parasitic infections affect persons living in developed countries, including America. Zoonotic diseases, i.e.

---

[20] Schmidt, GD and Roberts, LS., Foundations of Parasitology (4th ed). USA: Times Mirror/Mosby College Publishers, 1989.
[21] For a brief history of human parasitology, visit the site: http://cmr.asm.org/cgi/content/full/15/4/595. Further information can also be found at: http://www.alternative-doctor.com/allergies/parasites.htm

those transmitted from animals, are often caused by parasites, and infected people can even experience symptoms so severe as to be life-threatening.

Food can become contaminated if livestock, i.e. cows and pigs, are infected with parasites such as cryptosporidium and trichinella. People can acquire trichinellosis by ingesting trichinella-infected, undercooked meats. Cryptosporidiosis can be passed to humans if orchards or water sources near cow pastures become contaminated by infected bovine faeces; or if tainted fruit is consumed without being washed adequately beforehand.

In addition, pets too can act as parasite hosts and pass them on to humans. Young animals, such as puppies and kittens, are more likely to be infected with Ascaris and hookworms. According to official CDC data:

'Trichomonas is the most common parasitic infection in the USA, accounting for an estimated 7.4 million cases per year. Giardia and cryptosporidium are estimated to cause two million and 300,000 infections respectively in the US annually. Cryptosporidiosis is the most frequent cause of recreational water-related disease outbreaks in the US, causing multiple outbreaks each year. There are an estimated 1.5 million new toxoplasma infections and 400 to 4,000 cases of congenital toxoplasmosis in the US each year; 1.26 million persons in this country [US] have ocular involvement due to toxoplasmosis; and toxoplasmosis is the third leading cause of deaths due to food-borne illnesses (375+ deaths).[22]'

In the EU, the European Food Safety Authority (EFSA) was set up in January 2002 following a series of food crises, which have hardly subsided since then: mad cow/ sheep/goat disease, foot-and-mouth disease, bird flu and so on. In its latest report, the EFSA says the most commonly reported zoonotic infections in humans in the EU are, by far: '… those caused by bacterial zoonotic agents that can be shed by asymptomatic farm animals: the 2004 data indicates salmonellosis (192,703 reported cases) and campylobacterosis (183.961) – followed by yersiniosis (10,381), human listeriosis (1,267), parasitic zoonoses is 2,349 (trichinellosis, toxoplasmosis and echinococcosis put together). Compared to the main bacterial food-borne infections mentioned above (395,455 put together), reported human cases of 'classic' zoonoses are relatively low: brucellosis (1,337), tuberculosis due to M. bovis (86) and rabies (two imported).'

---

[22] The CDC's A-Z index listing of Parasitic diseases can be accessed at:
http://www.cdc.gov/ncidod/dpd/parasites/index.htm

It is important to bear in mind that official reports give only an indication of the situation in the European Community or the US due to serious under-detection and under-reporting, which varies by country or state.

But perhaps even harder to accept is that the parasites within you are infected by their own parasites in turn – parasites within parasites! The story is endless. For an enlightening exposition on the nature of symbiotic, as well as parasitic endobiotic relationships, (microorganisms living within other organisms) Dr Peter Schneider's article: 'Prof. Enderlein's research in today's view. Can his research results be confirmed with modern techniques?'[23] is enlightening.

Parasites, thus, are everywhere and in their most pathogenic states cause havoc in body, mind and spirit, with doctors responding with a range of treatments intended to suppress the symptoms, while failing to attack their source – the parasites themselves.

So, what can we do about these parasites we carry? Dr. Hulda Clark, Ph.D., N.D., a naturopathic physician, has brought the issue of parasitically-caused diseases and other types of toxicity back into the spotlight in recent years, dealing with this subject at length in her book: 'The cure for all diseases.'[24] Clark describes various methodologies and procedures to cleanse the body from these nasty creatures. This is not the only herbal parasite cleanse that is used at the Da Vinci Centre, as sometimes other therapies are combined using Sanum remedies, homeopathics, other herbal formulas and bioresonance therapy.

At the Da Vinci Holistic Health Center, we use Bioresonance diagnostics to identify the specific parasites in question and can therefore design bespoke anti-parasite programmes. However, generally, we use the PARAFORM PLUS ONE (one capsule x 3 times daily, away from food) mentioned above, along with PARAFORM TINCTURE (2 teaspoons in the morning, in a little water away from food). Both of these can be taken together.[25]

---

[23] Schneider, P. Prof. Enderlein's Research in Today's View: Can his research results be confirmed with modern techniques? First published in the German language in the *SANUM-Post magazine* (56/2001) Semmelweis-Institut, Germany, 2001.

[24] Clark, HR. The Cure for All Diseases. San Diego, CA: New Century Press, 1995.
[25] www.worldwidehealthcenter.net

Now that we have completed the all-body cleanse, the parasite cleanse and the heavy metal detox, we can now move on to the liver and gallbladder flush. There is no reason why you cannot continue the heavy metal detox for 2-3 months as doing this for only 15 days is not enough to eliminate a serious load of heavy metals from the body. The parasite cleanse can be run for 30 days comfortably.

If you suffer from chronic constipation, then this is likely to harbour more parasites as they like the toxic environment. Use a natural herbal to help your constipation such as CSTFORM. This powerful herbal formula contains Cascara bark, Senna, Turkey rhubarb and Wahoo bark.

Now after the preparations and the basic detoxification protocols that you have been through, it is time to look at preparing for the gallstone cleanse. It is imperative that you have taken for 15-days before the gallbladder cleanse, either one litre of apple juice daily or the magnesium malate – 1 cap x 3 daily – this is very important to do in order to soften the stones in the gallbladder so that there is no chance of any getting stuck in the gallbladder ducts. If you have not taken the apple juice of magnesium malate, then please **DO NOT** begin the gallbladder cleanse for the reasons mentioned.

How do we remove gallstones without resorting to surgery?
Cleansing the liver of gallstones dramatically improves digestion, which is the basis of your whole health. You can expect your allergies to disappear, too, more with each cleanse you do! Incredibly, it also eliminates shoulder, upper arm, and upper back pain. You have more energy and an increased sense of well-being.

I have personally witnessed the removal of gallstones from hundreds of patients – some of them with gallbladder symptoms expelled many stones that did not even appear on ultrasound, probably because they were trapped in the liver and gallbladder ducts and were not sitting in the gallbladder where the radiologists usually look.

Most, however, did not have any symptoms at all, yet would flush out literally hundreds of stones – no exaggeration! One woman in her 50's had three scans and the radiologists found nothing. She had pains in the gall-bladder region for 20 years. When she did the gall bladder flush she removed 280 stones the first time around, and about 200 the second time!

Here's her first flush with the gallstones – the coins are there to indicate size ratios and are Cypriot.

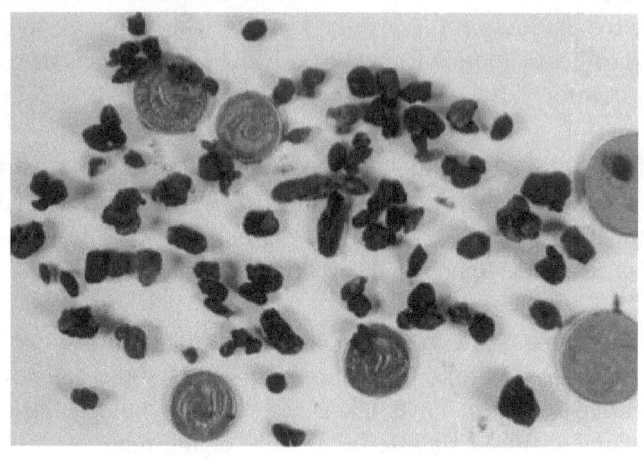

Gallbladder Stones Flushed Naturally

About a week before I did my first gall bladder flush (on myself) I went to see a friend who is an ultrasound specialist. He checked my gall bladder and found it as clean as a whistle. When I flushed a week later I removed 5 LARGE stones (about the size of a walnut), and about 150 smaller stones, including gravel – here is a photo of some of them:

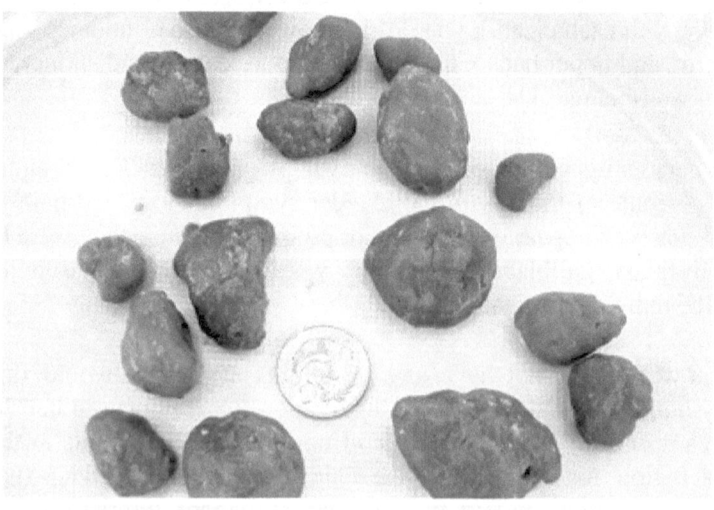

My stones on the first gallbladder flush

It is believed by many naturopathic doctors that EVERYONE has gallstones, even children, with all the junk food that they eat these days (but some less than others), and I have validated this many times in clinical practice.

The cleanse that I recommend below takes place within a period of less than 14 hours and can be done at home over the weekend. It is a harmless, pain-free and natural way of removing stones, without requiring invasive procedures such as surgery, laser, etc. Now that is a statement that will not be believed by the majority of general surgeons performing their gallbladder removals!

I had a personal experience of a 78-year old nun from a local convent here in Cyprus who was under my care for various health problems, including gallstones. She collected her stones in a jam- jar after her flush and took them to the surgeon at the local hospital here in Larnaca. His first reaction was, 'But that's impossible; you can only remove gallstones surgically or with a laser!' The nun looked at him in amazement and said, 'But Doctor, do you think I am lying to you?' whilst holding her rosary beads.

The surgeon adamantly persisted in his point of view whereby the nun said, 'OK Doctor, you scanned me about 3 weeks ago and you found stones and said that I require an operation. Is it possible that these stones disappeared by themselves?' He replied, 'No, this is not possible, once they are in the gallbladder they will stay there until they are removed, and yours were quite large, too.' The nun wisely replied, 'OK Doctor, if this is the case, then why don't you scan me again and let's see if they are in the gallbladder or in the jam jar?' So off they went to the ultrasound room, where he performed another scan – they emerged 30 minutes later after a thorough examination.

There were absolutely NO STONES in the gallbladder at all and now the surgeon looked really surprised. After a short silence, he perked up and said, 'I cannot see any stones now so this may have been a wrong diagnosis, but you certainly have quite a lot of sludge, so the operation should proceed.' The nun was flabbergasted and did not know what to say, but before leaving, they agreed to have the stones analyzed in the hospital lab – the results came back: 'GALLBLADDER STONES!'

The moral of this interesting story is: do not try to persuade your doctors and surgeons as there is a mindset akin to brainwashing where it is difficult for them to accept new concepts and treatments, particularly when they are based on the principles of Nature, who they are not too friendly with! Just keep the information to yourself – it is your health that you are trying to optimize, so why go through all the hassle of creating enemies with your doctor, who you may need on other occasions. Remember that many years ago, people and scientists were convinced that the world was flat, and it's ironic that there are still these believers in the 21st Century!

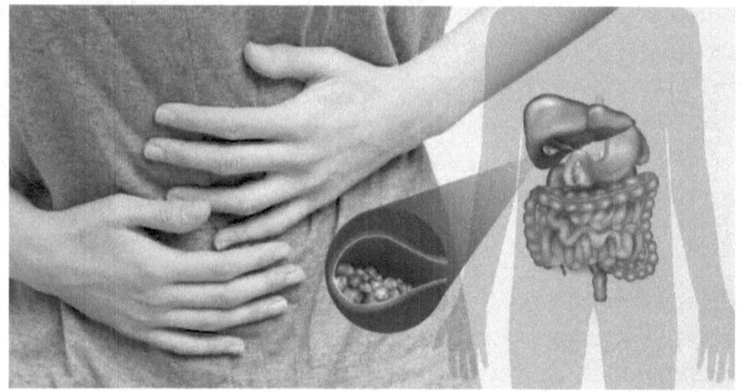

81

CHAPTER 6:

PREPARATIONS FOR THE GALLBLADDER FLUSH

OK, enough of the stories, let's proceed with the details of the gallbladder flush, beginning with the ingredients that you should first collect:

Apple juice (which is high in Malic acid and pectin); it acts as a solvent in the bile to weaken adhesions between solid globules, while softening the stones. This is crucial to the success of the procedure as it enables them to pass HARMLESSLY through the gall ducts.

The apple juice should be coarse, unfiltered and free of additives and preservatives – you will need to drink close to ONE LITRE (3-4 GLASSES) DAILY FOR 14 DAYS PRIOR TO THE FLUSH. In the worst-case scenario, if you cannot find fresh apples to juice, then you can use packaged apple juice, which should still contain these ingredients, but see if you can pick up some organic ones. An alternative to apple juice, which is just as effective, is taking Malic Acid in capsule form (magnesium malate). You will need to take one capsule, three times daily for 14 days before attempting the flush).

Four tablespoons of **Epsom salts** (magnesium sulphate). This allows magnesium to be absorbed into the bloodstream, therefore relaxing smooth muscles that surround the gallbladder ducts. This enables larger stones that may otherwise create spasms to pass through a relaxed bile duct. This is a very crucial part of the therapy and you CANNOT do the flush without taking these salts, which are freely available in most pharmacies. Ask for the B.P. variety for internal use, not those used for soaking in the bath – you will require about 70 grams per flush.

Half a cup of **Extra Virgin Olive Oil**, which stimulates the gall bladder and bile duct to contract powerfully, thus expelling the stones into the duodenum or small intestine. Once you drink the cup of olive oil and citrus fruits it enters the gut and the gallbladder which, detecting huge quantities of fat or oil, begins to go into spasm, expelling all the waste rubbish that has been stored for years.

At least a couple of large **grapefruits** (oranges will do if there are no grapefruits) mixed together with the juice of two fresh **lemons or limes**. The more acidic the juice, the faster the transit of the olive oil through the stomach and into the duodenum, which helps prevent or minimize nausea.

I have supervised hundreds of such cleanses using exactly this protocol that I am recommending here, without one patient suffering any harm whatsoever. But please follow the instructions carefully, and it must be said that you have ultimate responsibility, given that none of you are actual patients of mine.

On the day of the gallbladder flush there are some rules to follow:

1. Take no medications, vitamins or pills that you can do without on the day of the flush. They could prevent success.
2. Eat a NO-FAT breakfast and lunch such as cooked cereal with fruit, fruit juice, brown bread with a little honey (no butter, milk or margarine), baked potato or other vegetables with salt only.

2:00 PM – Do NOT drink or eat anything after 2:00 PM – only mineral water is fine, non-fizzy.

6:00 PM – Drink one serving (3/4 cup) of ice-cold Epsom salts. Mix one tablespoon Epsom salts into 3/4 cup cold water and stir well. You may add 1/8 teaspoon of vitamin C powder to improve the taste. You may drink a little water afterwards or rinse your mouth out. Epsom salts can also be mixed in with apple juice to make it taste nicer, or a few drops of lemon or lime can be added; or a little orange juice.

8:00 PM – Repeat the Epsom salt drink as above.

9:45 PM – Pour 1/2 mug (a large 10 oz. mug) of olive oil and squeeze 1/2 cup of orange or grapefruit juice into this, with the juice of two whole fresh lemons. Shake or stir hard until the oil and fruit juice mix thoroughly. Visit the bathroom now, shower, brush your teeth, go to the toilet etc. so that you are ready to lie down as soon as you have taken the olive oil mixture.

10:00 PM – Drink the olive oil and juice you have mixed. Drinking through a plastic straw helps it go down easier. Drink it standing up, not sitting or lying. You may use a little honey between sips to help it down. Try to drink it as quickly as you can, within 5 minutes.

TIPS: If you find it difficult drinking the olive oil mixture by itself, it is possible to mix it with prune juice or grape juice with a tablespoon of honey and put it in a blender for a minute or so.

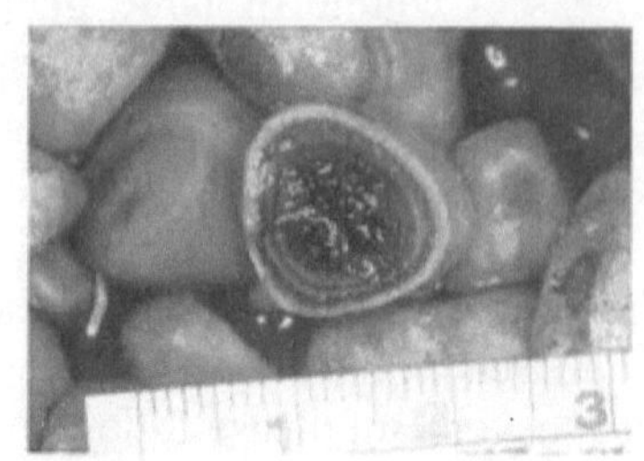

If you can obtain ozonated olive oil – maybe your naturopath has an ozonator and can make some ozonated olive oil for you – it may be better to use this as it will kill off any bacteria, parasites or other micro-organisms that may be lingering in the bile when it enters the intestine.

LIE DOWN IMMEDIATELY, ON YOUR RIGHT SIDE! You may fail to get stones out if you don't. The sooner you lie down, the more stones you will get out. Try to keep perfectly still for 20 minutes as the more you move the less stones your gallbladder will expel. You may feel a train of stones travelling along the bile ducts like marbles. There is no pain because the bile duct valves are open, thanks to the Epsom salts. GO TO SLEEP.

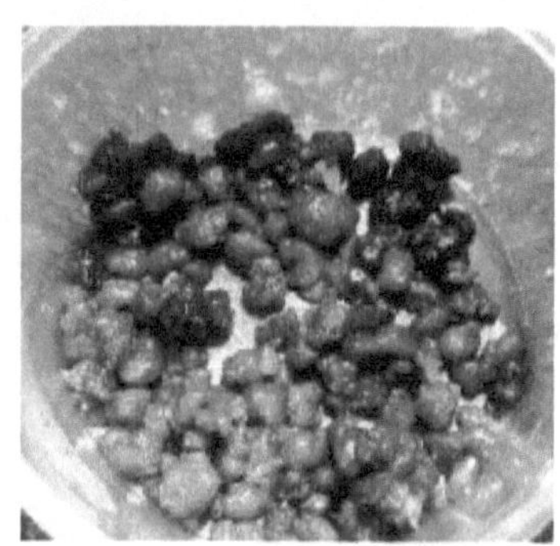

NEXT MORNING – upon awakening take another dose of Epsom salts. Drink 3/4 cup of the mixture. You may go back to bed. Don't drink this before 6:00 a.m.

2 HOURS LATER – take your 4th and last dose of Epsom salts. Drink 3/4 cup. You may again go back to bed and rest if you wish. Between the first and this dosage of Epsom salts, expect to frequent the toilet more often with diarrhea.

AFTER 2 MORE HOURS – you may begin to eat. Start with fruit juice or a carrot juice. Half an hour later eat some fruit. One hour later you may eat regular food but keep it light – salads, steamed vegetables, fruit, juices, etc. It's probably a good idea to drink some prune juice too as this will help to clear the gut.

BY SUPPER you should feel well. There are occasions when you may feel a little unwell for a couple of days, particularly if you have not done a liver flush before the gallbladder flush. Parasites in the liver can also cause symptoms to linger. Other times this may be due to stones and debris remaining in the colon and causing irritation and inflammation. Colon hydrotherapy or a good, deep enema can help this problem.

IN THE MORNING expect diarrhea. Try to catch the gallstones in a sieve placed on the toilet pan so that you can see them. If any of you have a digital camera, please take photos and send me a copy for my clinical archives.[26]

Most of the stones will be SOFT and green, breaking easily, or even dissolving. All these green stones are as soft as putty thanks to the malic acid in the apple juice and are mostly made of cholesterol. Some stones may be dark, near black in colour because of the bilirubin they contain. Other stones may be small and hard, made of calcium and oxalates (see image below). You may see all these types in one flush, but most of them will be the soft green ones made of cholesterol, as about 80% of the stones in the gallbladder are made of these.

A few days after the flush (maybe 10-15 days) stones from the rear of the liver will have travelled 'forward' towards the main bile ducts leaving the liver and fill the gall bladder again! This is why it is sometimes necessary to do up to 6 cleanses (perhaps one each month) in order to get rid of all the stones. If a cleanse produces no more stones, your liver can be considered to be in excellent condition!

---

[26] admin@docgeorge.com

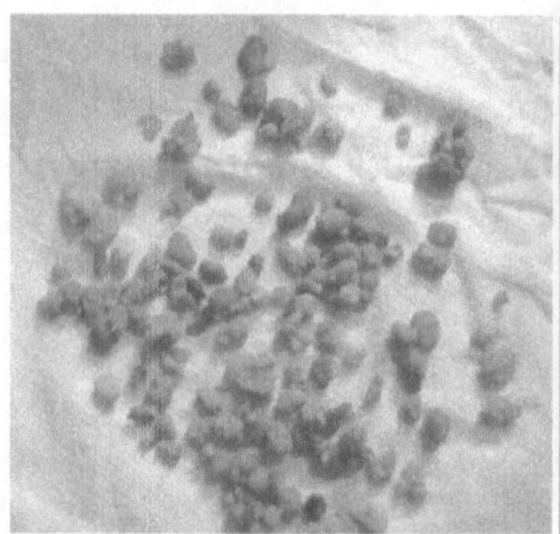 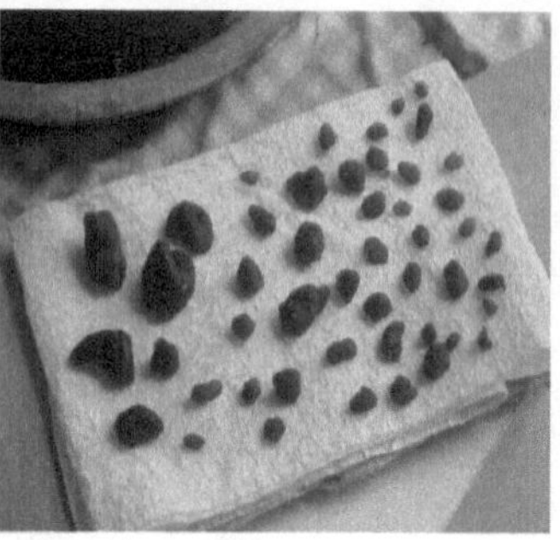

Helpful Tips

On rare occasions, some people may feel nauseous. This is related to the toxic bile leaving the gallbladder, causing discomfort and the feeling of wanting to vomit. There are a few things that may help in such cases:

- ❖ Taking one hydrochloric acid tablet at bedtime will help reduce any nausea during the night – these are sold in health food stores.
- ❖ If you tend to get nauseated from the oil, take 2 tablespoons of Aloe Vera juice after your doses of oil and citrus juice.
- ❖ Placing a hot water bottle over the liver area (under the right ribcage) during the night also helps relieve nausea.

Many people complete this procedure with minimal discomfort, and nearly everyone feels much better after completing it. Flushing the liver and gall bladder in the manner described (if the gall bladder is present) stimulates and cleanses these organs like no other process does.

Oftentimes, people suffering for years from gallstones, lack of appetite, biliousness, backaches, nausea, and a host of other complaints, will find gallstone-type objects in the stool the day following the flush. These objects are light to dark green in colour, very irregular in shape, gelatinous in texture, and of sizes varying from 'grape seed' size to 'cherry' size. If there seems to be many of these objects in the stool, the flush should be repeated in 2-4 weeks.

Complications of Gallstones

Choledocholithiasis occurs in 20% of patients with gallstones. *Common bile duct obstruction* may result, and may be partial or complete, continuous or intermittent. This may lead to jaundice and biliary-type pain.

In bad cases, *Acute pancreatitis* may occur as result of ampullary obstruction by a gallstone (30% - 75% of patients with acute pancreatitis have gallstones), or papillary stenosis.

Gallbladder cancer accounts for one third to one half of gallstone related death in USA. About 80% of patients with gallbladder cancer have stones, and 1% of patients with gallstones at autopsy have gallbladder cancer.

Cohort studies suggest that patients with symptomatic stones develop gallbladder cancer at higher rates than do patients with asymptomatic stones. Gallbladder cancer occurs in 50% of patients with a calcified gallbladder wall (porcelain gallbladder).

Homeopathic Remedies for Gallbladder Symptoms
There are several homeopathic remedies that can be used along with the gallbladder flush to help alleviate symptoms. Homeopathic remedies are generally freely available in most health food stores and are very safe to use at all ages.

The remedies suggested here should be either as a 6c or 30c potency – these can be taken between 2-4 times daily, depending on the severity of your symptoms. Here are the most common homeopathic remedies for helping with gallbladder symptoms:

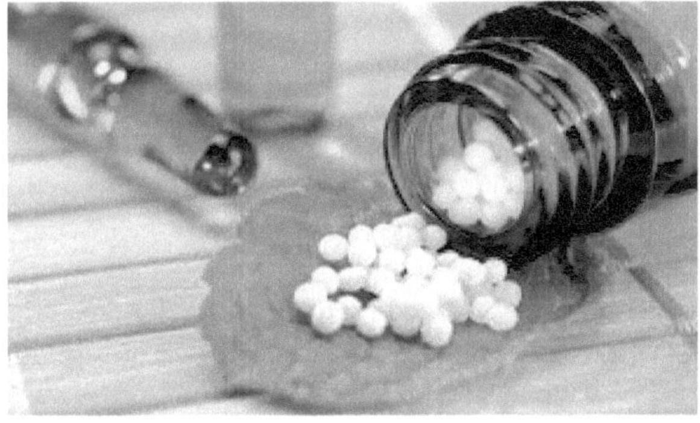

Berberis vulgaris – recommended for individuals whose symptoms include:

• Stitching pains that extend from the stomach area to the shoulder
• Twinges of sharp pain in the groin and pelvic area

• Increased pain when standing up or changing position
• Constipation

Calcarea carbonica – recommended for individuals whose symptoms include:

• Bloated or swollen stomach area, particularly on the right side
• Cutting pains and tenderness
• Pain worsens when standing or when tired, and pain improves when lying on one side
• Often fatigued and sluggish
• Excessive craving for sweets

Chelidonium majus – recommended for people who have the following symptoms:

• Pain that is located in the back, right shoulder and shoulder blade
• A distended abdomen
• Worse pain when moving
• If lying on the left with the legs drawn up helps alleviate pain
• Nausea, especially after eating fat or drinking cold beverages
• Exhaustion

Colocynthis – for people who suffer from the following symptoms:

• Sharp cramping pains causing a person to double over in pain
• Pain in the upper right abdomen that radiates into the shoulder
• Increased intensity of symptoms in the evening

Dioscorea – for individuals with the following symptoms:

• If pain from gallstones is lessened by bending backwards
• Pain from gallstones is worse when bending forward or lying flat
• Pain spread to the back, chest and arms
• Pain is worse in the evening and night

Lycopodium – this is a good, general remedy with people that have the following:

• Bloating and flatulence
• General abdominal discomfort

Nux vomica – this is a traditional tonic for gastrointestinal symptoms such as:

• Stitching pains in the right upper abdomen
• Digestive cramps
• Nausea
• Excessive fat cravings and stimulants such as caffeine
• Irritability

In addition to these homeopathics, if you are in pain or distressed then RESCUE REMEDY is a good remedy that will help to remove a lot of the tension and stress and help you relax quickly.

It may also be worthwhile taking a natural heavy metal chelator that can remove toxic metals and other xenobiotics from the body – one of the most researched is called HMD™[27]

Further Detox Regimes
Apart from the detox protocols that we have already mentioned, there are a few more detox regimes that would be worth knowing about. If you have an opportunity to use these, they are good for preventing gallbladder stones in the future. They also help to eliminate toxins from the body and prevent their accumulation, which could cause other degenerative diseases over time.

The Infamous Coffee Enema – The Detox Secret!
If you are feeling lousy during the 15-DADD, there is one thing that can give immediate relief - you will be surprised and maybe shocked to hear it. It's a coffee enema. Yes, that's having a cup of coffee, but not by mouth!

The use of coffee in enemas for detoxification purposes is well known. It is a common remedy that has been used by holistic and alternative medicine professionals for many years. It is commonly used in cancer clinics that treat cancer using natural methods.

---

[27] www.detoxmetals.com

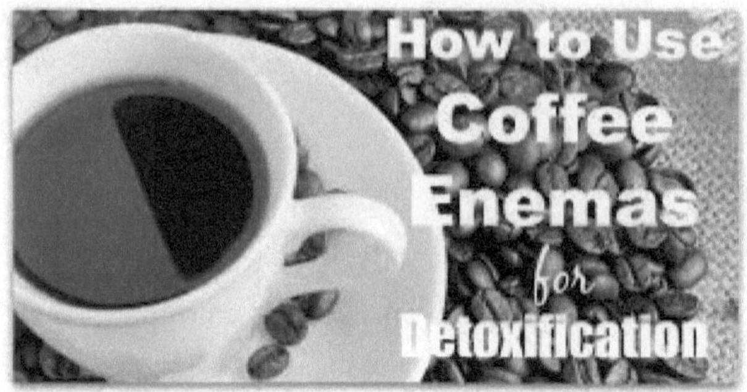

How does the coffee enema work?

The effects of a coffee enema are different than a saline or herbal enema. The caffeine, theophylline and theobromine – which are all phytonutrients found in coffee beans – combine to stimulate the relaxation of smooth muscles, causing dilation of blood vessels and bile ducts.

The effects of having a coffee enema are not the same as drinking coffee. In terms of their physiological effect, studies have shown that the rectal instillation of fluids will stimulate gallbladder contraction and emptying, with the elimination of the many toxins that the bile contains. This was reported as far back as 1929 by Garbat and Jacobi.[28]

There is a direct communication of veins from the rectal area to the liver called the enterohepatic circulation or Portal Vein system. This means that the coffee is absorbed into the haemorrhoidal vein, then taken up to the liver by the portal vein where it stimulates the liver to produce more bile with all its processed toxins, and moves this bile out toward the small intestine for elimination.

---

[28] Garbat and Jacobi. Secretion of bile in response to rectal installations. *Archives of Internal Medicine*, Volume 44, pp. 455-462, 1929.

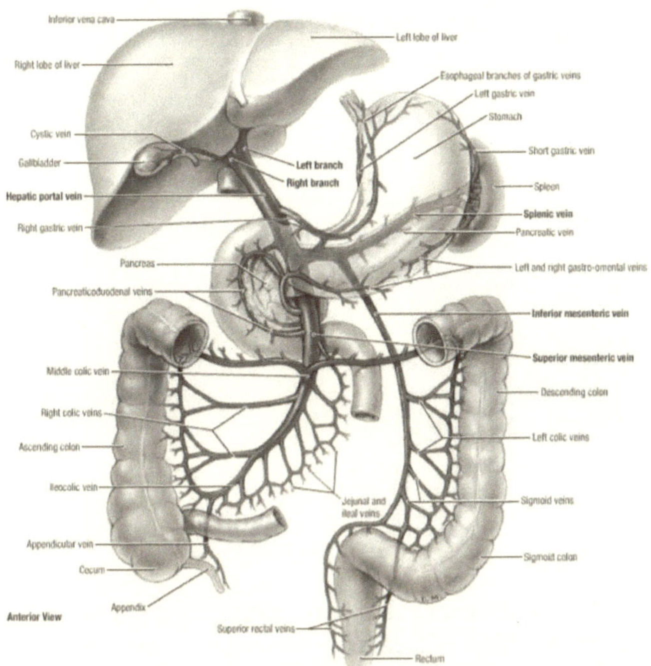

The coffee also contains certain alkaloids, which stimulate the production of glutathione-S-transferase (GT) in the gut, one of the main detoxification enzymes produced by the liver. Research has shown that the levels of GT can increase by about 600% when coffee enemas are administered. Moreover, the enzymes in coffee known as palmitates further help the liver to eliminate the toxins contained in bile acid. With the bile ducts dilated, bile carries toxins away to the gastro-intestinal tract. Simultaneously, peristaltic activity is encouraged because of the flooding of the lower colon – further eliminating toxic loads.

The benefits of increasing quantities of GT in the gut are:

- ❖ GT binds bilirubin and its glucuronides so that they can be eliminated from the liver cells.
- ❖ GT blocks and detoxifies carcinogens, which require oxidation or reduction to be activated. Its catalytic function produces a protective effect against many chemical carcinogens.
- ❖ GT forms a covalent bond with nearly all free radical substances which is the precondition for their elimination from the body.

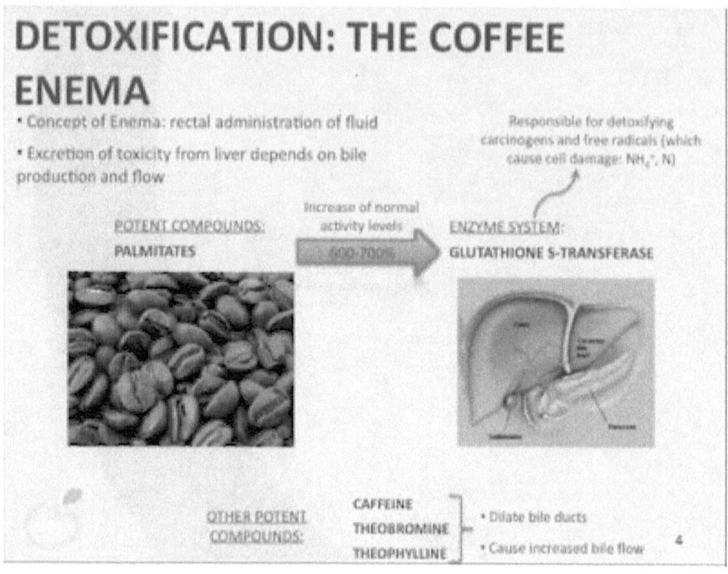

In 1981, Dr. Lee Wattenberg and his colleagues showed that substances found in coffee - kahweol and cafestol palmitate - promote the activity of a key enzyme system, glutathione S-transferase, above the norm. This system detoxifies a vast array of electrophiles from the bloodstream and, per Gar Hildenbrand of the Gerson Institute, *"must be regarded as an important mechanism for carcinogen detoxification."* This enzyme group is responsible for neutralizing free radicals, the harmful chemicals now commonly implicated in the initiation of cancer. In mice, for example, these systems are enhanced 600% in the liver and 700% in the bowel when coffee beans are added to the mice's diet.

Dr. Peter Lechner, who is investigating the Gerson method at the Landeskrankenhaus of Graz, Austria, has reported that *"coffee enemas have a definite effect on the colon which can be observed with an endoscope."*

As many of you have never had an enema in your life, let alone a coffee enema, here are a few guidelines to follow to make the experience a pleasant one…

Preparing the Coffee Enema Formula
It's quite simple to prepare a coffee enema – it's probably better to make a certain quantity for say 8 enemas and store this in a glass bottle in the refrigerator. Below is how to make the coffee concentrate, enough for 8 enemas:

1. Boil 2 litres of purified water
2. Add 340 grams of ground organic coffee
3. Simmer for 1/2 hour
4. Cool, then strain
5. Reconstitute to 2 litres
6. Put into 2 x 1-litre glass bottles (milk or juice bottles) and mark bottles at 250mls with marker

How do you use a coffee enema?
1. Take 250mls of coffee concentrate
2. Add enough warm, purified water to make up to one litre
3. Hang the enema kit (usually a plastic bag of 1-1 ½ litres with a narrow hose attached with a rubber insert at the end and a tap or clip to control the flow) on a tap or door with the douche bag approximately 40-60 cm (1-2 feet) above where your body will be. You could try hanging it on a window or door knob – use a metal hanger or improvise by tying a length of string onto the enema bag and tying this somewhere.
4. Make sure the valve tap is closed
5. Pour the 1 litre diluted coffee enema into the douche container
6. Open the tap to clear all air out of the tubing, being careful not to lose coffee, then turn the valve off
7. Place a blanket and towel on the floor
8. Lubricate the tip of the catheter with KY-Jelly or similar gel-lubricant (do not use Vaseline)
9. Lie on your right side, insert the tip of the catheter (approx 2-3 inches) with both legs drawn close to the abdomen to allow the fluid to run into the bowel slowly. You can also try lying on your back - see below for other positions.

Use the tap to turn off during use (i.e. if you get cramping or the feeling that you are full).

It's important to try to retain the fluid for as long as possible up to 15 minutes – it may be that initially you cannot hold the fluid for longer than 2-3 minutes. This is OK but try every time to hold it for longer periods of time to get the maximum absorption and maximal benefits.

Do this once a day after your normal bowel motion throughout the 15-day ADD. Remember you are using the coffee enema as a way of cleaning the liver and toxic gallbladder, not as a means of stimulating peristalsis and bowel evacuation, even though it can have this advantage as well.

What position should you use?

You have a few choices as far as positions are concerned. Here are some examples:

- ❖ The left side position: Lie on your left side. Bend your right leg (upper leg) toward your chest. Keep your left leg straight. This position should be comfortable while giving good access to your anus.
- ❖ Doggie style (knee chest) position: Kneel on your elbows and knees with your head down and your buttocks high in the air. You might even want to put your chest to the floor.
- ❖ On your back: Lie on your back with your knees bent. Your knees should be together while your feet are separate. This should allow good access to your anus from below.

<u>Note:</u> It is possible to undergo an enema on a toilet, however in this position the body is almost forced to expel. You will most likely have trouble holding an enema while seated.

Temperature is important when administering an enema – 102 degrees Fahrenheit or 37 degrees centigrade is about body temperature. If the water is colder or hotter than this then it may cause spasms and cramping of the intestine, leading to rapid expulsion and pain.

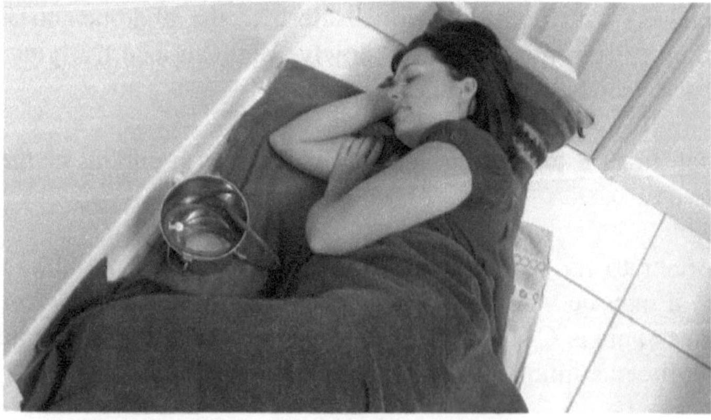

Administering Your First Enema

Prepare your enema, hang it in the appropriate position (about 1-2 feet above your anus) and take up your chosen position. The clamp should be on the enema tubing close to your hand, so you can have easy control over it with one hand.

Lubricate your anus with the KY Jelly or similar – you don't need too much, but it would be good to apply a little lubricant to the tip of the enema tube too.

Now push down to relax and open the sphincter muscle at the anus – take a deep breath if this helps. You should not really feel the tube entering when the anus is relaxed and there should certainly be no pain.

Once the tube is inside, turn on the flow slowly and begin filling the colon. Stay calm and concentrate on the water filling your colon. Once you feel pressure, see how much you can feel comfortable with and then turn off the flow. Stay in this position for as long as you can so that the coffee can be fully absorbed.

If you feel the need to evacuate, try and stay still for a few seconds – usually the feeling goes away as the colon relaxes.

When it is time to evacuate, simply get up slowly with the tube intact and sit on the toilet – remove the tube slowly and evacuate.

As soon as you have evacuated, take up position again and refill your colon and again hold the coffee in for as long as you can.

Repeat this procedure until all the coffee has been used up.

After completing your enema, you can use some hydrogen peroxide in water to sanitize your equipment or any other antiseptic that you may have available. When you have completed washing the bag, simply hang it up to dry to avoid any mould growth.

Note: Enema bags should be used only by one person and should not be shared, much like a toothbrush.

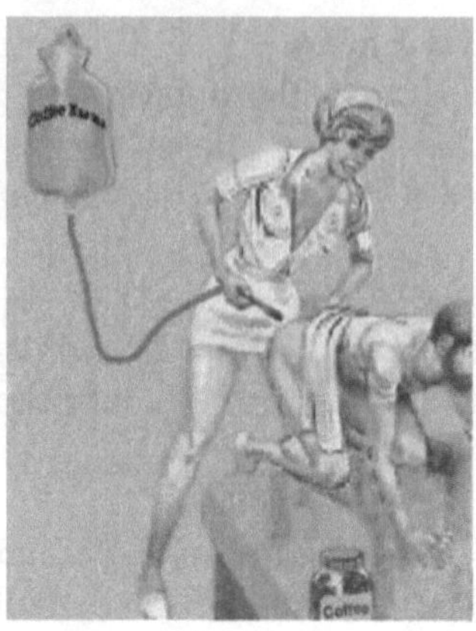

Skin Brushing

The body is much like a large lake with many tiny streams running from it. The 'streams' help to drain the toxins from the body. These tiny 'streams' join up to form what is known as the lymphatic system of the body, and it does just that – removes toxins. One of the best and simplest ways of stimulating lymphatic drainage is with a technique called SKIN BRUSHING. It stimulates the movement of lymphatic fluid in the lymph vessels and helps to break down congestion in areas where the lymph flow has become sluggish and toxins have collected.

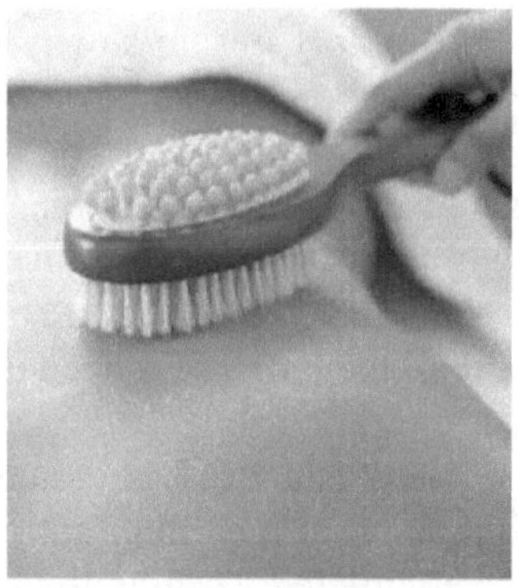

This is also an excellent technique to remove unsightly cellulite in women – a condition in which stasis of lymph fluid has accumulated excess proteins, fats and waste materials in certain areas of the body. This eventually results in puckered skin, alterations to connective tissue and distortions of the natural body shape.

You must put aside 5 minutes of your day and practice this wonderful technique, particularly during the 15-day detoxification programme. Before your bathe in the morning and evening, brush your skin all over with a natural-fibre brush (one that looks like a clothes brush but made of natural as opposed to synthetic fibres). You can begin from the shoulders and work down over the whole body, except the head. Use long, smooth strokes and work from the shoulders downwards to the waist, and then from the feet upwards to the waist. You only need to go over the skin once, every time you do it. Press as firmly as you feel comfortable with – as you become fitter you will be able to use more pressure.

You will be utterly amazed at how much junk and toxins are eliminated through the pores of skin, using this method. After all, the skin is one of the largest detoxification organs of the body, spreading out over 2 square metres – that's a large organ. If the other detoxification organs are congested, such as the liver, kidneys and gut (constipation), then you can bet your life that the skin will be working overtime.

To test the efficacy of this method, every time you skin brush, simply wipe your skin with a flannel and hang it up in the bathroom. After a few days of doing this, the smell of the flannel will be quite revolting due to the quantity of waste products that have come directly through the skin's surface.

Detox-Breathing Exercise
This powerful breathing exercise will help you eliminate the toxins you are releasing and strengthen and tone your entire system.

CAUTION: Do not use if you have a heart condition, high blood pressure, epilepsy, a hernia or if you have any ear, nose or eye problems.

1. Inhale slowly and deeply. Don't overstrain in any way.
2. Exhale briskly, as if you were sneezing. As you do, become aware of your abdomen, which will naturally tighten and flatten as you exhale.
3. Inhale naturally and exhale briskly again.

Continue this cycle for as long as you feel comfortable. It is very energetic, so you may not be able to manage more than a minute to begin with. Do it regularly throughout your weekend and notice how you improve.

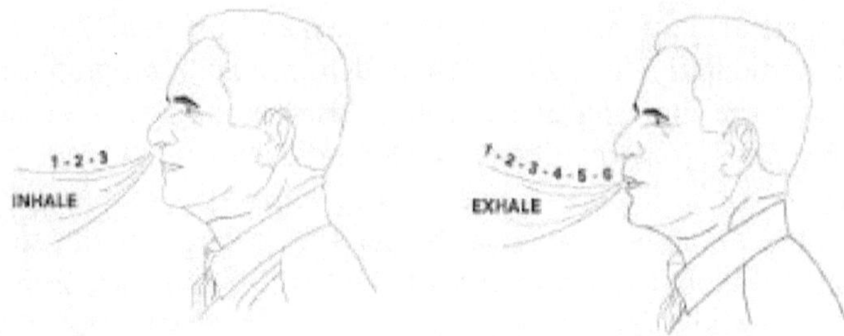

When you finish, return to normal breathing. Take notice of how you feel.

You could also try a good massage session: manual lymphatic drainage is particularly useful while detoxing because it supports the lymphatic system. But any massage will do you good (ask your therapist to use detoxing oils if you're having aromatherapy).

Detox 'Visualization'
After your detox-breathing, spend some time doing some visualization exercises.

Sit either on a straight-backed chair or on the floor.

Check your body to ensure you aren't holding on to tension, especially in the jaws, shoulders, legs and buttocks.

Now focus on your breathing. Don't try to change it – just be aware of it. Notice how you breathe in and how you hold your breath for a moment before exhaling. Then pause again before you inhale. It's a four-step process.

Continue breathing like this and if your mind starts to wander, don't get annoyed with yourself – just gently bring it back.

Imagine you're exhaling toxic thoughts and emotions from your body and mind, and inhaling new, exciting energy and possibilities.

Now become aware of your body – of your buttocks sitting on the floor or chair; of your head balancing on your neck; of your shoulders relaxed and heavy.

Now become aware of the world around you: the sounds, the temperature. Slowly and gently open your eyes and return to normal consciousness.

Sit for a few minutes. Drink some water before getting up. You should now be in a very relaxed and tranquil state.

Epsom Salts Bath
Before turning in for an early night, you're going to have a thorough skin-brushing session and then take an Epsom-salts bath. This induces a lot of perspiration, so you can sweat out lots of the toxins you are starting to release.

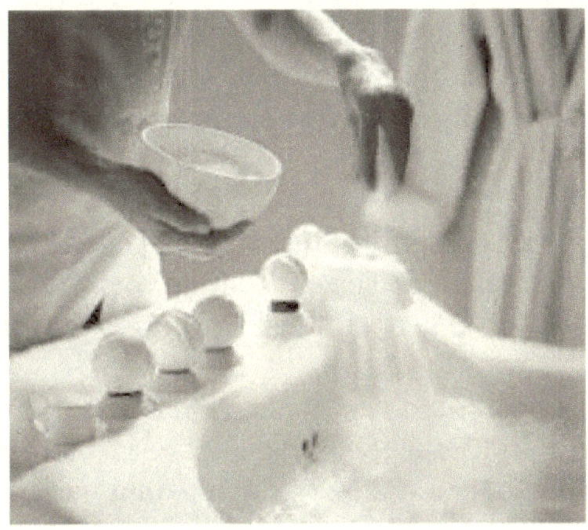

CAUTION: Avoid taking this bath if you have heart trouble, are diabetic or feel tired and weak. Instead, you can substitute with a mineral bath or the cider vinegar bath described below.

Dissolve the amount of Epsom salts according to your weight into a warm bath – which shouldn't be too hot - as follows:

- ❖ Up to 60 lbs (28 kg) – ½ cup
- ❖ 60 – 100 lbs (28 – 45 kg) – 1 cup
- ❖ 100 – 150 lbs (45 – 70 kg) – 1 ½ cups
- ❖ 150 – 200 lbs (70 – 90 kg) – 2 cups

For every additional 50 lbs (20 kg) bodyweight, add an extra ½ cup. One cup weighs about 8oz or ½ lb or 0.25 kg.

Get in and relax for about 20 minutes. Visualise all the toxins coming out from your pores and dissolving in the water. Drink a hot herbal tea (thyme or peppermint) to increase the sweating and replace any fluids you lose. You can prepare this in a flask before you get into the bath or have your partner bring it in.

Get out carefully as you may feel light-headed. Don't rub your body; just swathe yourself in large, warm towels and go to bed, making sure your feet are wrapped up warmly. You'll probably go straight to sleep.

Cider Vinegar Bath
Again, plan to get to bed early. Skin brush thoroughly (you should be an expert by now). Add two cups of apple cider vinegar to your warm bath. Make sure that the water is not too hot. Get in and relax for about 15 minutes. This bath is deeply detoxifying. Pat yourself dry and go to bed.

Sauna or Steam Bath
This may be considered an optional luxury as opposed to an essential, but if you have access to a sauna or steam room at your local leisure centre or health club, then take advantage of it during your 15-day detox.

If you have serious health problems such as diabetes, valvar heart disease, high blood pressure or advanced arteriosclerosis, seek medical advice first before you march off to the sauna – you don't want it to exacerbate existing health problems.

Saunas are excellent for opening the pores of the skin and allowing toxins to leave the body quickly. It is recommended that you take a short warm shower followed by 10 - 15 minutes in the sauna, then a 30-second cold plunge or shower. It is a good idea to take a few minutes' rest now while the body's physiology returns to normal after the initial 'shock'. Take another 10-15 minutes in the sauna once you are used to the process, followed by a cool shower or plunge, then a rest. If you can afford a massage now, you will really be indulging yourself, your skin and your health.

When in the sauna, stay on the bottom bench first until your body acclimatises, then you can think about moving to the upper bench. Drink plenty of mineral water - your body needs it. And do not eat for an hour before or after the sauna.

The Theory of Autointoxication

The compelling suspicion that a stagnant bowel filled with putrefying matter can leak out and become a source of infection for the rest of the body was first suggested by the ancient Egyptians. In the 19th century, this became known as 'The theory of autointoxication – self poisoning from one's own retained wastes.' This idea has been enthusiastically embraced by every subsequent generation. One of the main causes is constipation.

Constipation

Constipation has done more to provide the health profession with an obvious solution to un-diagnosable ailments than any other simple complaint. It is defined as 'The difficult or infrequent passage of faeces' and it is associated with the presence of dry, hardened stools.

Constipation is a national pastime and slow bowels are more common today than years previous. For one thing, people not only ate better 100 years ago, they were more active and got out doors more.

When the bowels slow down, toxins are not eliminated but are reabsorbed and carried back to the liver for recycling and elimination. Reabsorbed bile salts have been linked to increased cholesterol levels. Therefore, high cholesterol is a major precursor of constipation. Also, when the bowels get slow and toxin levels increase, the pathogenic microorganisms grow to out-number the normal flora, causing dysbiosis.

Although friendly bowel flora such as Acidophilus (small intestine) and Bifidobacteria (colon) are needed to correct this, it is the clogged bowels that are the major problem. When the bowels move again, everything else will fall into order.

Our endocrine glands (which control metabolism), are also involved since it is our thyroid that controls metabolism and metabolism affects how our bowels function. In this way, constipation can be seen as a symptom of hypothyroidism. Low body temperatures (a symptom of hypothyroidism) are very common today –although they are not 'normal' – as many authors have reported.

Intestinal toxaemia (a form of blood poisoning), is caused by the absorption of bacteria and their toxins through the intestinal wall. The large intestine (colon) is the most prolific source of bacterial contamination in the entire body. Thirty-six toxic substances have been isolated from the human colon, including such compounds as indole, skatole, phenol and cresol.

When these kinds of toxins are passing through the intestinal wall, they can enter the lymphatic or portal system and be directly transported to the liver. Temporary increases in the toxic load of the liver occur during periods of stagnation in the colon. Any prolongation of this state will impede the detoxification and bacteria-killing function of the liver. The importance of this function cannot be overlooked when one realizes that blood from the intestinal tract enters the liver before it is delivered to the tissues of the body.

An overburdened liver, which cannot handle the toxic load from the intestine, transfers the task of detoxification onto another organ - the kidney. Unfortunately, the kidney is not able to reduce the amount and kind of toxins that enter the liver, nor can it detoxify them as efficiently as the liver. The toxins that the kidneys do not remove from the blood increase circulating body-toxin levels.

The Oxford Dictionary defines constipation as, *'Irregular and difficult defecation.'* The question is, *'What is a regular bowel movement when there is no norm?'* Regularity becomes a meaningless expression when some people have a bowel movement regularly every Sunday morning, while others regularly empty their bowels after every meal.

Defecation is a reflex action, stimulated by distension of the rectum with faeces. It is under voluntary control in adults and normally takes place only when time and circumstances are suitable. The presence of food in the stomach stimulates a reflex action called peristalsis, which moves food residue into and along the colon. Mass peristalsis gives us the feeling that we need to empty our bowels. This reflex action usually occurs after the first meal of the day but can also be stimulated by only drinking some liquid on rising.

If the call to defecate is persistently neglected, the reflex mechanism becomes less sensitive and constipation can result. This is likely to happen when there are time constraints causing hurry and stress (stress ceases peristaltic action in the colon).

Some healthy people don't defecate every day and do not have any discomfort. Many others open their bowels every day with excruciating agony – passing dark, rock hard, compacted stools. Both cases would be considered constipated.

Ideally, one should defecate as many times as we have a proper meal, usually 3 times per day. Although the main rule is that we should have a bowel movement at least once a day. The stool should be fibrous, light in colour, float in the water, break up easily and cause no pain or discomfort to pass – in fact no toilet paper should be needed. Pain or discomfort whilst passing hard or dry stool at less than daily intervals can be considered as constipation. Many people have suffered heart attacks as a result of vigorous efforts to have a bowel movement as continuous efforts to evacuate material from the rectum increases the heart rate, blood pressure and respiration.

Referred to essentially as a Western disease, constipation is virtually unheard of among third world people adhering to traditional fibre-rich diets. Constipation is implicated in many Western diseases such as diverticulosis, obesity, varicose veins, cancer of the colon and rectum, appendicitis and haemorrhoids. These are all very rare in undeveloped countries.

Whatever the causes of constipation, it is important that you should try to use some gentle herbal formulas and supplements in order to help the transit time of the gut.

At the Da Vinci Center, I use the following formulations to help my patients. They can all be combined if required and the dosages can vary depending on the condition and the patient:[29]

1. <u>CONSTFORM</u>
2. <u>COLFORM</u>
3. <u>OXYGUT</u>

Nature Needs Some Help and Urgently

❖ In the U.S., approximately 80 million people suffer from bowel problems.
❖ 100-120,000 a year lose their lives – usually from bowel cancer.
❖ Colon cancer is the second leading killer in the Western World.
❖ Behind these statistics are also those saved by colostomies (surgical removal of the large intestine), which in the US only approximately 250.000 people a year receive.

---

[29] www.worldwidehealthcenter.net

❖ In UK and the rest of Europe, the numbers are more or less the same.

Bowel experts all over the world now agree that poor bowel management is the root of most health problems. The faulty Western commercialized diet is the focal point of the problem. A diet high in meat, white sugar, white flour, fat, and low in dietary fibre and water is believed to be connected with constipation.

The root of the problem is clearly indicated by laxative sales, estimated at *600–800 million dollars a year.*

Laxatives aggravate the problem of constipation by interfering with the colon's ability to eliminate normally on its own. The chemicals within laxatives irritate and stimulate the colon to abnormally contract, to expel the irritating substances. In addition, the oral route of administration is the least optimal method for evacuation of the colon because crucial digestive processes occurring in the stomach and small intestine are interfered with. Most laxatives and purgatives precipitate dehydration.

Hippocrates took the view of not disturbing and messing up the entire peptic system with harsh laxatives, as the problem lies at the extreme end of this same system. Standard enemas, even highly recommended as first aid, only cleanse the rectum and last portion of the colon, missing out most of the large intestine.

Colon Hydrotherapy is an extended and more complete form of an enema. This method extends beyond the rectum to cleanse the entire colon and offers greater therapeutic benefits. It addresses the cause or source of the constipation problem. Other methods treat only the symptoms and provide temporary relief of the problem.

Why constipated? The biggest reasons? Dietary (lack of natural dietary fibre and consumption of devitalized foods, especially white sugar, white flour and all their by-products); neglecting the urge to eliminate; dehydration (too little water); stress; too little exercise (sitting for long hours); abuse of stimulants and drugs; irregular hours (work – rest, wake – asleep) and pathological conditions.

The most common signs and symptoms due to an impacted, constipated colon are:

- ❖ Infrequent or difficult bowel movements; hard compacted stools and low stool weight
- ❖ Tiredness, fatigue, lethargy, lack of energy, poor concentration and irritability
- ❖ Bloating and flatulence
- ❖ Headaches, mental depression or dullness
- ❖ Irritable Bowel Syndrome, diverticulosis, colitis, leaky gut, cancer of the bowel, Crohn's Disease, appendicitis, hiatus hernia
- ❖ Malabsorption, bad breath and a coated tongue
- ❖ Haemorrhoids, varicose veins, obesity and cellulite

Colon Hydrotherapy

Colon Hydrotherapy is one of the most powerful and effective ways of cleansing and detoxifying our entire system. The mucous membrane of the large intestine is the first and most important defence system against toxic substances (followed by the liver, the lymph system, lungs and the skin), thus a very important part of the body's immune system.

As I outlined above, nearly all doctors and practitioners of natural medicine take the view that most disease originates in an unhealthy colon.

Exogenous toxins such as poor nutrition, sterilized and denatured foods, environmental toxins and poisons, abuse of medicines and narcotics as well endogenous toxins from emotional conflicts and stress, clog detoxifying channels on an on-going basis.

Having three bowel movements a day does not negate the fact that after years of dietary indiscretion, a gradual build-up of mucus and undigested foods begin to form in the lining of the colon.

Dehydration and stagnation occur. Our bodies are being poisoned by these toxic substances which can cause inflammation, damage the intestinal wall and cells, and intoxicate the nerves and glands. These toxins can also be absorbed through the walls of the colon into the blood and lymph; ultimately to into the cells and tissues. The resulting toxaemia can become a chronic condition, but for most of us it creates erratic conditions in the body that we call *disease*.

Indications for Colon Hydrotherapy

Colon Hydrotherapy may be undertaken with the approval of a physician or health care professional for: acute faecal impaction, Crohn's disease, diverticulitis, mucous colitis and during the first four months of pregnancy when it may alleviate morning sickness. Other indications include: abdominal discomfort, acne, bad breath, constipation, candida overgrowth (yeast syndrome), carbohydrate indigestion, celiac disease, cellulite, diarrhoea, digestive problems, diverticulosis, eczema, excessive mucus, flatulence (gas), IBS (irritable bowel syndrome), nausea, stomach bloating, sluggish atonic colon, mild to moderate haemorrhoids, intestinal toxaemia, parasites and worms, spastic colon, shingles, systemic toxicity, thrush and varicose veins.

Colon Hydrotherapy can also be a part of a holistic approach in conditions where the immune system is compromised, such as: allergies, arthritis, cancer, chronic fatigue, Epstein-Barre, gout, lupus, migraine headaches, MS (multiple sclerosis), psoriasis, rheumatoid arthritis, sciatica, sinusitis etc.

Colon Hydrotherapy is also found to be beneficial in conjunction with medical procedures such as: pre-and post-surgery, barium x-ray, bowel and stomach examinations.

It can be used as a preventative measure; athletes have opted for colon therapy to improve metabolic efficiency; it can be very beneficial when suffering from colds and influenza, life-style change, weight loss programmes and travelling.

It is of utmost importance for elderly and handicapped persons, in fasting and cleansing programmes and when working through emotional issues.

However, it is contraindicated for any of the following conditions: gastrointestinal bleeding, cancer of the colon or rectum, anal fissure or fistula, abdominal hernia, acute haemorrhoids, severe cardiac disease, renal insufficiency, pregnancy after four months, or up to six months after colon or rectal surgery.

What is Colon Hydrotherapy?
Colon Hydrotherapy is a gentle and safe method of cleansing the large intestine (colon) from toxic waste material, including gas, accumulated faecal matter, parasites and mucus deposits. This is achieved by introducing a continuous flow of purified water into the colon, accompanied by abdominal massage – which helps to break up impaction and remove collected, stagnating stool throughout the colon, thereby stimulating the channels of elimination into removing stored toxins from different areas of the body.

This process is painless, easy and odourless. The water and waste are run out through a transparent waste tube so that the amount, form and type can be observed and judged. Contrary to traditional enemas, the treatment is thorough and cleanses the entire colon. The treatment lasts about 45 minutes to one hour and is totally hygienic – all equipment is disposable, and the cleansing is always performed by a qualified colon hydrotherapist. The physical goals of each session are to hydrate the system, remove waste, stimulate peristalsis, and rehabilitate nerves, muscles, glands, circulatory and immune systems.

Before Colon Hydrotherapy, eat lightly during the previous day. On the day of the cleanse do not consume any food or water (liquid) for at least 2 hours before the treatment. Your abdomen will be massaged, and you will need to urinate less, if at all, during the session. Bring a t-shirt so that you feel comfortable.

Heavy Metal Detoxification
We will discuss this in a separate chapter on toxicity, but we can briefly mention that heavy metals such as arsenic, aluminum, antimony, cadmium, lead, mercury and uranium are insidious in today's world. There is probably not a person on this planet that does not have some of these in their system, leading to heavy metal toxicity, which is the cause of many illnesses.

The early signs of heavy metal poisoning are vague or often attributed to other diseases. These include headaches, fatigue, muscle pain, indigestion, tremors, constipation, anemia, indigestion and tremors. Mild toxicity symptoms include impaired memory and distorted thinking ability. Severe toxicity can lead to death.

Hair mineral analysis is a convenient but often unreliable screening test. The most accurate measurement is by blood analysis of actual toxin levels within the red blood cells. Many toxic metals tend to accumulate inside the cell, where most of the damage is done.

One of the safest and most effective ways to remove heavy metal toxicity is to use a natural heavy metal chelating therapy named 'The HMD Ultimate Detox Pack[30]. The main formulation that mobilizes the metals is called

---

[30] https://www.detoxmetals.com/product/hmd-ultimate-detox-pack/

HMD™ – you will need to take 45 drops, three times a day shortly before meals, in some water or juice.

In addition, there are two other drainage remedies that can be taken along with the HMD™, and are part of the HMD Ultimate Detox:

ORGANIC CHLORELLA (475 mg) for absorbing the stray heavy metals that may get reabsorbed from the gut. Recommended adult dosage: 2 tabs three times per day.

ORGANIC LAVAGE combines several organic herbs that help to clean the blood and help the kidneys, liver and lymphatic system to open and drain the toxins out of the body. Recommended adult dosage: 25 drops x 3 daily for 3-6 months, along with the HMD™ and chlorella.

Lung & Lymphatic Cleanse
The lymphatic system is the garbage collector; the internal vacuum cleaner sucking up metabolic garbage, toxins and excess fluid from the extracellular fluid of every organ. If this flow is impaired, the fluid becomes thick and toxic. The parts of the body that rely on it for elimination become less efficient and sluggish as they fill with their own waste. This otherwise life-sustaining system now becomes a breeding ground for infection. When the fluid enters the bloodstream, as is part of the normal process, infection can spread to any organ or part of the body. Many viruses, bacteria and parasites stay locked within the lymphatic system when these conditions are present. The result: physical ailments, degenerative disease, the hastening of the aging process and even death!

The lymphatic system acts as a secondary circulatory system, except that it collaborates with white blood cells in the lymph nodes to protect the body from being infected by cancer cells, fungi, viruses or bacteria. It is a system of thin tubes that runs throughout the body, called 'lymph vessels.'

Unlike the circulatory system, the lymphatic system is not closed and has no central pump. It is not under pressure and only moves because of exercise or muscle contraction. When the lymphatic system is congested, the cells become deprived of oxygen, affecting the body's ability to rid itself of its own waste material. Over time, other body systems that rely on the lymphatic system for waste removal will also become compromised, setting the stage for pain and disease.

Swollen glands, with which most of us are familiar, are symptomatic of blocked lymph nodes, which indicate a breakdown in the mechanical functioning of the lymphatic system.

Other symptoms/diseases of congested lymphatics				
Allergies	Chronic sinusitis	Heart disease	Eczema & other skin conditions	Loss of energy
Prostatitis	Fibrocystic disease	Chronic fatigue	Repetitive parasitic infections	MS
Oedema	Lupus erythromatosis	Inflammation	High blood pressure	Viral infections
Puffy eyes	Bacterial infections	Low back pain	Loss of energy	Cancer
Ear or balance problems	Arthritis	Headaches	Cellulite	Excessive sweating

Detoxification Exercises
Rebound exercise, using a small rebounder or trampoline is so efficient in stimulating the lymph flow that Dr. C. Samuel West calls it 'Lymphocizing.' This is truly a fabulous way to move the lymphatic fluid, as well as exercise the lungs and other systems of the body. Every house should have a rebounder! The up and down rhythmic bouncing causes all the one-way valves to open and close simultaneously, increasing lymph flow as much as fifteen times!

Aerobics exercise, which is widely associated with cardiovascular health, also helps cleanse the lungs. During active and intense exercise, forced expiratory volume of the lungs' oxygen exchange capacity is increased, and 'dead air' normally trapped within the small alveoli of the lungs is expelled in exchange for fresh air. It is therefore important to exercise in non-polluted areas.

Breathing exercises combined with physical activity increase the action of lymphatic cleansing. Jumping jacks work well when you synchronize your breathing with the movement of your legs and arms. When you are walking, or jumping on a trampoline, inhale four times and exhale four times – one breath with each jump, but slowly. Move your arms and legs each time you take a small breath. Inhale through your nose and exhale through your nose or mouth - swing your arms forward and back in time with each pace and breathe with each step.

Kidney & Blood Cleanse

To optimize kidney cleansing, drinking one quart of pure filtered water per day for every 50 pounds of body weight is one of the absolute basic foundations for anti-aging. If you are in good health, try drinking 10 to15 glasses of water daily. It is best to limit your intake to filtered or bottled water.

The right kind of water is especially important. Distillation is the process in which water is boiled, evaporated and the vapor condensed. Distilled water is devoid of dissolved minerals and is thus able to actively absorb toxic substances from the body and eliminate them. Drinking distilled water during detoxification for a short period (less than 4 weeks), helps the body to eliminate unwanted minerals. Once this is accomplished, distilled water consumption should be discontinued.

Long term use of distilled water can be dangerous because of the rapid loss of sodium, potassium, chloride and trace minerals which can inevitably lead to multiple mineral deficiencies. Furthermore, distilled water can potentially over-acidify the body. When exposed to air, distilled water absorbs the atmospheric carbon dioxide, which becomes acidic with a pH of 5.8. – normal drinking water should be slightly alkaline with a pH of 7.2-7.4.

The ideal water for long-term human consumption should be slightly alkaline and contain minerals such as calcium and magnesium. Water filtered through reverse osmosis tends to be neutral and is recommended for long term consumption. Water filtered through a solid charcoal filter is slightly alkaline. Make sure that the filter you choose is of good quality and removes pollutants and parasites such as cryptosporidium. The best type of filter to do this is a reverse osmosis filter.

Some of the herbs which can help cleanse and support the kidneys include Juniper berries, Parsley root, Marshmallow root, Golden Seal root, Uva Ursi leaves, Lobelia herb, Dandelion, Gravel root and Ginger root.

Infrared Heat Therapy

Infrared rays are energy waves produced by the sun and are part of the electromagnetic spectrum, each section of which has energy of different wavelengths. Other waves include visible light (the rainbow colours), microwaves, ultraviolet rays and X-rays.

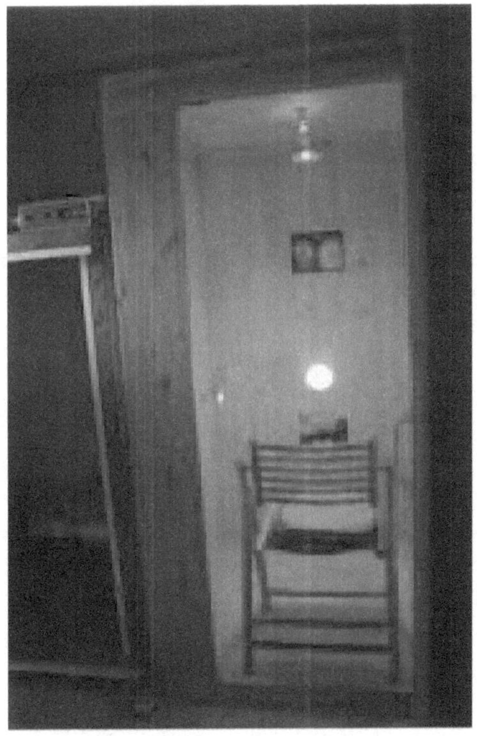

Da Vinci Center's Infrared Sauna

Infrared energy is a radiant form of heat. It heats objects directly through conversion, without having to heat the airspace between. This infrared heat, in the form of special lamps, pads or mats, is routinely used by physical and massage therapists and chiropractors.

The benefits of infrared therapy are numerous: improvements in microvascular circulation of blood and lymph; enhancement of tissue fluid exchange; relaxation of muscles; improvement in flexibility; deep cleansing of soft tissues with efficient removal of toxins and waste products; the improvement of fibroblast functions for connective tissue repair; acceleration of cellular metabolism; stimulation and support of immune system functions; reduction of physical and psychological stress and fatigue. In fact, there are hardly any medical conditions that do not benefit from infrared heat therapy, in particular infrared sauna therapy.

In an infrared sauna, our bodies absorb most of the infrared radiation directed onto our skin. The heat here produces more than three times the sweat volume produced by conventional saunas, at much lower temperatures. Additionally, infrared saunas can be used by heart-disease patients because they operate at a relatively low temperature and humidity, allowing easier toleration of the treatment.

The sweat produced from an infrared sauna is also fattier (oily) because the heat penetrates deeply into the fat layers of the body. This property allows for the removal of heavy metal toxins that accumulate because of sluggish elimination or high exposure. Many clinics' detoxification programs, including the Da Vinci Natural Health Centre, use an infrared sauna for mercury and other toxin elimination. Heavy metals become mobilized and eliminated through sweat, stool, urine, and hair.

The Sauna Experience
Drink four ounces of water before entering a sauna and eight or more ounces afterwards. Add sea salt to your diet, and two tablespoons (or about 10 tablets) of kelp daily, especially if your water is mineral-free. Remove metal jewellery before entering a sauna, as it may become very hot.

Preheat an infrared electric light sauna for 10-15 minutes, or you may enter as soon as you turn it on. It need not become hotter than $115f$. When it reaches $115f$, open the door slightly so the sauna stays at this temperature.

Preheat a traditional sauna to $150f$. With a far infrared sauna, enter as soon as you turn it on, or preheat for 10-15 minutes. A far infrared sauna need not be hotter than about $130f$. When it reaches $130f$, open the door slightly to continue receiving the rays without it getting any hotter.

You may wear light clothing in a traditional sauna. Clothing is not used in infrared or far infrared saunas. The beneficial rays are best received directly on the skin.

Use a small towel to wipe off sweat. Sit on another small towel. Have a third towel on the floor to avoid slipping. Meditate or relax. Talking or working are not recommended while in a sauna.

To enhance the effects of a sauna session, you may visualize absorbing the heat and energy through every pore. You may also visualize releasing toxins as you sweat. Deep, slow breathing and sitting up straight are also helpful. Sound therapy, such as listening to low tones, is also excellent.

In an infrared electric light sauna, with lamps on one side, turn every few minutes to heat the body evenly. Sit on a stool or a chair without a back. Face the lamps, turn to the side and around to the back. Avoid touching the hot lamps. Looking at the lamps is not harmful but is not recommended. Do not let water, a towel or clothing touch the hot lamps. One will not get a tan in an infrared sauna, though the skin may redden for an hour afterwards.

Finishing Up
How long you remain in a sauna depends on your health condition and how long you have used saunas. Body temperature should not increase more than four degrees. Your pulse should not increase more than 50% of your resting pulse. Begin with 15 minutes if you are ill. If your heart begins to race, sweating stops or you feel very faint, end the session immediately. Sixty minutes is the maximum time.

When finished, take a shower. It may be warm or cool, but not hot. Clean the body with a skin brush or loofa in the shower. Brush all over, even your face and hair. It may be painful at first. However, it soon feels wonderful. Skin brushing enhances the cleansing effect of the sauna.

Avoid soap if possible, as you should be very clean. Soap can leave a film and clog the pores. Use shampoo and conditioner only if needed. Most contain chemicals toxic to the body. Also, skip most oils, lotions and creams. These also contain chemicals that may clog the pores. Rinse out the towels used in the sauna, so they will be ready for your next sauna session.

After showering, drink eight or more ounces of water. Sit for at least 10 minutes. These simple steps allow the body to reap the full benefit of the sauna experience.

Supervision and Safety

Supervision during a sauna therapy program is always best, and essential if one has a chronic condition. The presence of an attendant or friend is also most helpful.

Removing drugs from tissue storage may cause flashbacks or temporary drug effects, the same as when you took the drug. If you have used LSD or other psychotropic drugs, have an attendant close by, as a few have experienced flashbacks or even full-blown LSD trips.

However, saunas are quite safe for most people, providing one follows the procedures above. If debilitated or very heat sensitive, begin with less time in the sauna. Always consult a health professional if one has multiple sclerosis, a serious heart condition or other chronic illness.

Pregnant women and children under five should avoid saunas. Young children must be accompanied by an adult. Continue prescribed medication while taking saunas, unless directed otherwise.

Use a sauna twice a week to twice a day. If one is very debilitated, begin with once a week. Work up to daily use as you are able to do so. When beginning, stay inside only 20-25 minutes. Many people do not sweat easily. Instead, their bodies overheat, and they tolerate less time in the sauna.

In a few weeks to a few months, most people acclimate to sweating and can easily regulate their body temperature. Sweating often increases a lot over a few months. The more one relaxes, the more one will sweat.

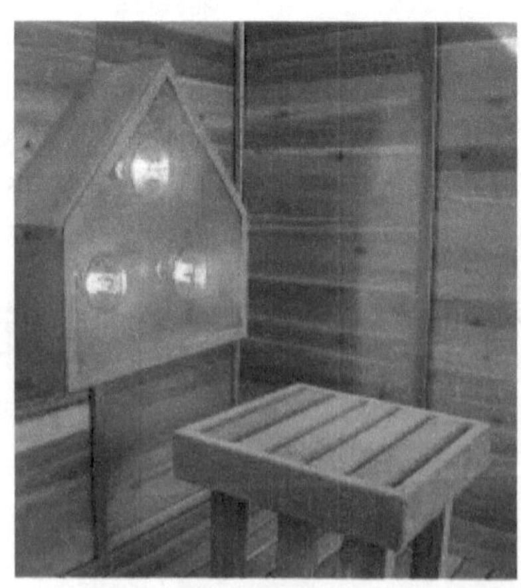

Healing Reactions

Healing reactions are temporary symptoms that occur as toxic substances are eliminated, and chronic infections heal. Symptoms vary from mild odours, tastes or rashes to periods of fatigue, bowel changes, aches, pains or headaches.

Almost everyone has some chronic infections. These may flare up as they are healed due to repeated sauna use. Usually only rest and natural remedies are needed to help infections resolve faster.

Emotional healing also takes place, especially with the use of infrared electric light saunas. Memories may arise consciously or, at times, in dreams. Temporary anxiety or other emotional states may occur and usually pass quickly. Some are directly related to the elimination of toxic substances. Others are associated with emotional clearing.

Almost all healing symptoms are benign and will pass quickly. Consult a knowledgeable practitioner if any cause concern.

An Integrated Healing Program

A healthful lifestyle and an integrated healing program greatly enhance the results of sauna therapy. Rest several times during the day, eat natural foods, breathe deeply and exercise a little each day.

Reduce your exposure to toxic chemicals at home and at work. Toxic products range from pesticides and insecticides to solvents, body care products, paints, cleaners, new carpeting and toxic building materials.
A specific diet for your metabolic type and a supplementary nutrient program based on a properly performed hair mineral analysis are also most helpful, and essential when body chemistry is far out of balance.

Ionic Footbath Therapy

This mode of therapy uses an electrical device for external detoxification. At the Da Vinci Holistic Health Centre we use the Focus Ionic Footbath (http://hymbas.com).

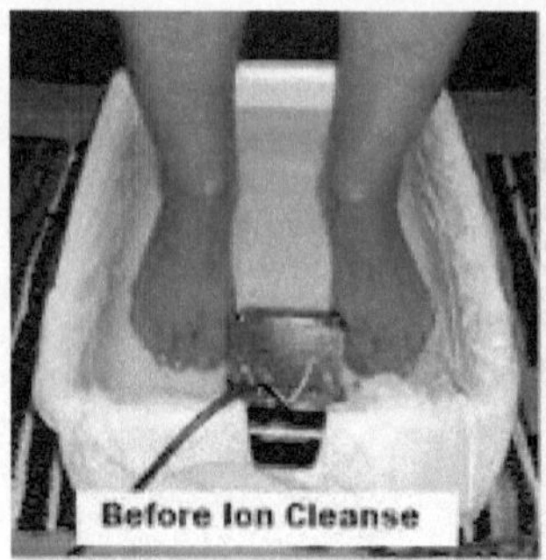

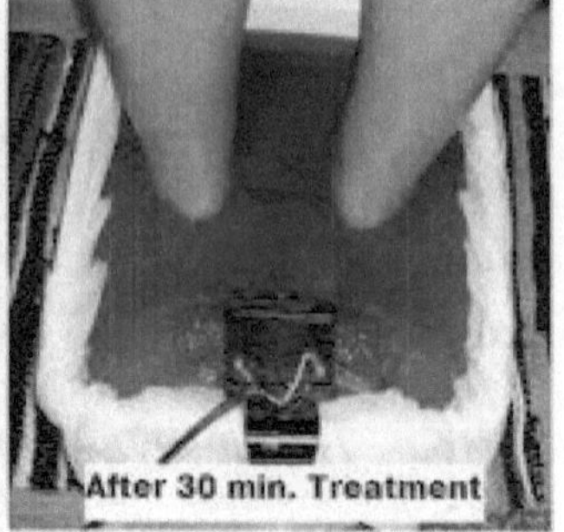

How do these devices work?

Firstly, you need to know what an ion is: a charged atom or molecule that has gained or lost an electron, thus creating an electromagnetic field capable of neutralizing opposing-charged particles, such as toxins, in the human body. With a foot spa, the main control unit delivers an electrical current through the ionizer probe placed in the water of the footbath.

The low-level direct current to the probe causes the water and salt to generate positively and negatively-charged ions by separating the oxygen and hydrogen components of water. The Bio-Body Cleanser allows the positive and negative ions to travel through the body (ion channels) and attach themselves to toxic substances with the opposite charge. Since most toxins in our bodies are in the form of positive ions, they will be neutralized and cleansed by the negative ions produced by the ionic footbath therapy.

With a constant flow of negative ions being produced in the water, this also raises the user's pH to a more alkaline state. This is important because most people live in an acid state; their bodies contain an excess of hydrogen ions, and their pH is lower than 7.45 – a normal value. Such individuals need exposure to higher concentrations of negatively-charged ions to shift their pH to a more balanced acid-alkaline state.

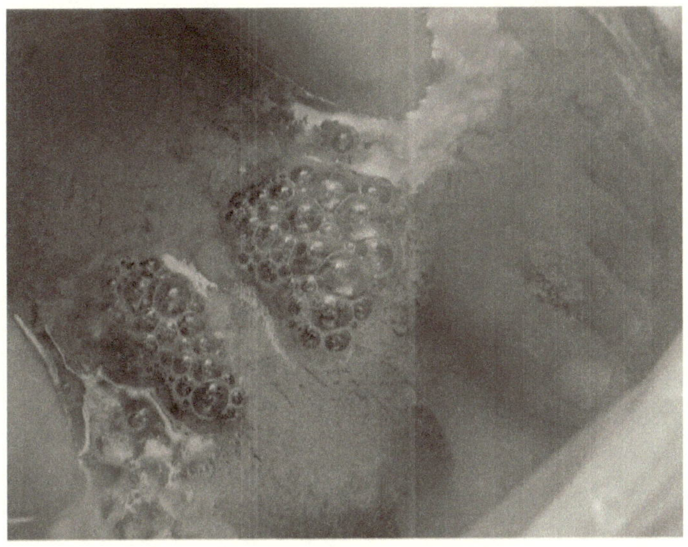

Toxins in the ionizing footbath

Putting it all together

It makes a lot of sense to avoid the factors that cause gallstones in the first place, otherwise they are likely to form again.

It's not clear what causes gallstones to form. Doctors think gallstones may result when:

- **Your bile contains too much cholesterol.** Normally, your bile contains enough chemicals to dissolve the cholesterol excreted by your liver. But if your liver excretes more cholesterol than your bile can dissolve, the excess cholesterol may form into crystals and eventually into stones.

-

- **Your bile contains too much bilirubin.** Bilirubin is a chemical that's produced when your body breaks down red blood cells. Certain conditions cause your liver to make too much bilirubin, including liver cirrhosis, biliary tract infections and certain blood disorders. The excess bilirubin contributes to gallstone formation.

- **Your gallbladder doesn't empty correctly.** If your gallbladder doesn't empty completely or often enough, bile may become very concentrated and this contributes to the formation of gallstones.

Factors that may increase your risk of gallstones include:

- Being female – twice as many women get gallstones than men
- Being age 60 or older
- Being overweight or obese – this will double the chances of getting gallstones
- Being pregnant
- Eating a high-fat diet – mostly saturated fats
- Eating a high-cholesterol diet
- Eating a low-fibre diet
- Having a family history of gallstones
- Having diabetes
- Losing weight very quickly
- Taking some cholesterol-lowering medications such as statins
- Taking medications that contain oestrogen, such as hormone therapy drugs (HRT) and contraceptive pills
- Taking certain antibiotics such as ceftriaxone

So, we can see from the list above that there are certain lifestyle changes that can help, such as:

1. Eating a diet that is low in cholesterol and saturated fats – the best way of doing this is to eat more fish and seafood, and less meat.
2. Adding more fibre into our diets by eating plenty of salads, vegetables, fruits and whole meal cereals, as opposed to refined.
3. Keep your weight down by avoiding junk foods, sweets, high sugar foods, trans fats from processed foods and exercising regularly.

Where can I begin?
A good starting point is to avoid the things mentioned above and begin making the lifestyle changes towards a healthier lifestyle.

Given that all of us are quite toxic from the food, water and pollutants we take into our bodies, as well as the toxins that are produced internally due to stress and negative emotions, it would be good to detoxify by following the instructions in the chapter on Detoxification.

The would begin with an alkaline detoxification diet, eating plenty of salads, vegetables, fruits, vegetable juices, herbal teas and a few nuts. Take a herbal remedy such as <u>LAVAGE</u> to help the detoxification organs. Please remember that you would need to take either apple juice daily for two weeks, as the malic acid it contains helps to soften the stones. However, if you suspect that you may have Candida, then best to take <u>MAGNESIUM MALATE</u> – one cap x 3 daily, with food.

In parallel, you can take some herbal remedies to clear some of the parasites that have accumulated – <u>PARAFORM PLUS ONE</u> and <u>PARAFORM TINCTURE</u> are a couple that you can take.

If you suspect having toxic metals, then you can take the <u>HMD ULTIMATE DETOX PACK</u> that has already been discussed in another chapter. If you wish to find out if you have toxic metals, then taking a <u>HAIR MINERAL ANALYSIS</u>[31] is a good way of finding out.

After the two weeks of detoxification, then you are ready to proceed to the Gallbladder cleanse described in the previous chapter.

If you have been drinking heavily, or eating lots of fatty and sweet foods, then it would be best to take <u>HEPATO PLUS</u> for at least a couple of months or more to help the liver to clean and strengthen. <u>DTXFORM TINCTURE</u> also helps to detoxify the liver.[32]

Make certain that you avoid all foods that you are intolerant to as these will cause a lot of inflammation in the body. You can ask a Bioresonance practitioner if they can treat these foods for you.

Do not forget to also detoxify emotionally as negative emotions can prevent us from reaching our full potential.

Emotional Detox

Let's look at some of the common emotions that can prevent you from moving forward, growing and optimizing your health.

Problems in the gallbladder indicate trouble dealing with feelings and,

---

[31] https://www.detoxmetals.com/hmd-hair-test-testing/
[32] www.worldwidehealthcenter.com

particularly, clarifying them." What is my place? Am I being granted recognition for what I do?" The person goes through fits of anger but will not express his feelings. For this reason, he does not get rid of his bile and, instead, he stores it.

The person who suffers from gallbladder problems is someone who feels invaded by someone close and is unable to express his feelings.

When I feel anger or aggressiveness, I feel I may attack the other person. For this reason, the sympathetic nervous system gets ready for it, gets ready to fight and resorts to adrenalin. The person loses his mind. People who store anger have chronic tension on their shoulders, neck and arms.

There are three solutions to deal with anger:

1. To play the denial game and pretend everything is OK, and that the cause has been resolved, when it clearly has not.

This "solution" does not actually solve anything and makes the person accumulate anger, something that could cause problems later.

2. To ventilate emotions proactively by playing sports such as rugby, boxing, karate and the like. The extreme would be to become violent and aggressive to others without provocation.

This "solution" resolves the effect but not the cause, and makes the person increasingly more dependent on that violent activity, which then becomes a permanent "support" and entering a negative cycle of meaningless aggression.

3. To introspect and look deeply inside us and become aware of our feelings, even if this means that we should cry.

This solution resolves the cause and dissipates the emotions. The person can allow their anger to ventilate in a more constructive and meaningful way through awareness and observation of themselves. The propensity for anger also will diminish.

So, anger seems to be directly associated to gallbladder problems and incorporates the liver too.

Another author and researcher, Louise Hay, mentioned that gallstones could be tied to bitterness, hard thoughts, condemning or pride. Over the years, these unexpressed emotions could solidify into gallstones. And if it causes a lot of pain and inflammation, it also represents the seething anger.

What could be causing us to be so bitter? Could we find in our hearts to forgive? Everyone tries to live their lives the best way using what they've been given and conditioned. They may hurt us in the process. And we can see that holding on to that resentment and bitterness is not doing us any good.

The person could be now enjoying life and oblivious to our suffering. And here we are, suffering by ourselves. Is it worth it?

So, let go of the anger and soften your heart – simply forgive. In forgiving the other person, we also forgive ourselves and "let go" of the negative energy that will be stored in our organs causing harm.

We forgive ourselves for making the mistake of trusting and loving the person. It's time to learn from the mistake and betrayal and move on in life. Look around - there is still a lot of goodness in the world. There are many other people who are kind and love us – let us move on with these people and allow the hurt and stored emotions to dissipate – let another Higher Power take care of the justice that is due.

CHAPTER 7:

SIMPLE RULES TO AVOID GALLSTONES

There are several things that we can change in life in order to live healthier and avoid gallstones from forming.

1. Cleanse your liver twice a year

After you have eliminated all your gallstones through a series of liver cleanses, it is best to cleanse the liver twice a year. I recommend to my patients to clean their livers every time they go through the 15-day Da Vinci Alkaline detoxification diet, which is basically every 6 months.

The best date for a liver cleanse is about one week before the seasons change. So 15th March, 15th June, 15th September and 15th December. I usually run mine in March and September when there are plenty of fruits and vegetables around and the weather is still warm.

2. Avoid overeating

Overindulging in foods is one of the major causes of gallstones. The golden rule is really to get up from the table with a little more room to eat a little more. Also, taking a day per week to stay on liquid foods such as soups, juices, herbal teas and plenty of water will help keep the gastrointestinal system in peak shape. Avoiding quick energy foods such as sugar, sweets, chocolate, colas and the like – all the refined foods which will lead to gallstones.

3. Reduce alcohol intake

Alcohol is a liquefied sugar, as it is converted to sugar very quickly in the body. A couple of glasses of wine and the liver will begin storing fatty deposits in the liver, which can lead to gallstones.

4. Drink plenty of water

The body produces over a litre of bile per day, so requires plenty of water for this function as well as many others. The body cannot store water as it can fat, so drinking at least 1.5 – 2 litres per day (or more in hot climates) is essential to overall health and keeping gallstones at bay.

5. Eat regular meals on time

The body has numerous circadian rhythms that regulate important functions of the body. Eating regular meals conditions the body to produce the correct amounts of digestive juices for each meal. Skipping meals and eating at different times will disrupt the cycles of bile production by the liver cells, leading to the formation of gallstones.

6. Avoid processed and refined foods

All processed and refined foods will cause imbalances in the production of bile that will lead to gallstones. Try eating more fish and seafood, as opposed to meat which is full of saturated fats. Low fat foods will also impair bile secretions, causing stagnation of bile leading to gallstones.

7. Sleeping adequately

Lack of sleep will lead to a gradual deterioration of body processes. The most powerful rejuvenation taking place in the body take place a little before midnight, during the initial cycles of REM sleep.

8. Controlling overwork stress

Many people get trapped in a cycle of overworking in order to have the adrenaline rushes that seem to keep them going. This cycle will eventually exhaust the liver and immune system and lead to many illnesses, including gallstones.

9. Regular exercise

Regular exercise will help us to increase our capacity to digest food, eliminate physical and emotional toxins and generally strengthen our body to deal with all the stresses of daily life. A sedentary process will slow down the blood flow to the liver and lead to gallstones.

10. Sunlight daily

Regular exposure to sunlight has been shown to lower cholesterol levels which is one of the major causes of gallstones.

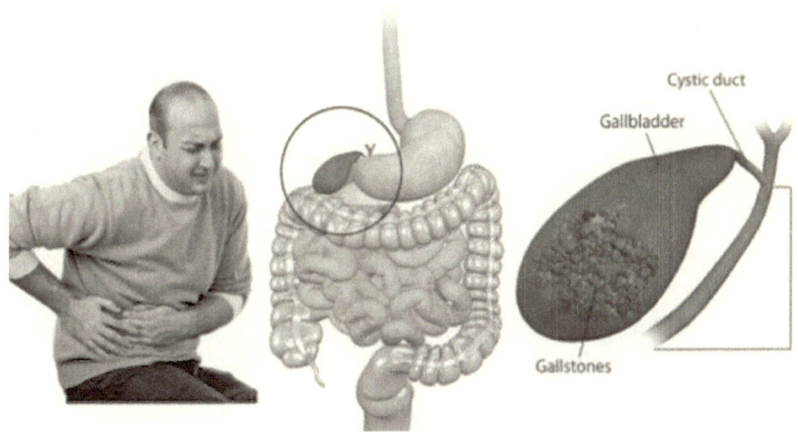

CHAPTER 8: CASE HISTORIES

CASE HISTORY: Mrs. K, Age 30

Main presenting problem: Acute Gallbladder Colic due to stone obstruction

Medical diagnosis:

This patient presented with acute pains in the liver area which reached the shoulder area. An ultrasound scan taken 8.9.08, showed: "the gallbladder is distended, with a length of 8.5 cm and a transverse diameter of 5.3 cm. There are no large gallstones evident, but there are echogenic contents in the dependent part of the gallbladder, suggestive of bile sludge (on a previous examination, small calculi were identified within the gallbladder). There is mild dilation of the common bile duct, which measures 9mm in diameter, down to the level of the ampulla of vater. The features are in keeping with a partial obstruction to the distal gallbladder, probably as a result of microlithiasis, or bile sludge."

In addition, she presented with blood analysis taken 4.9.08 showing the following elevated enzymes:

ALT - (alanine aminotransferase) - was previously called SGPT is more specific for liver damage. The ALT is an enzyme that is produced in the liver cells (hepatocytes) therefore it is more specific for liver disease than some of the other enzymes. It is generally increased in situations where there is damage to the liver cell membranes. All types of liver inflammation can cause raised ALT. Her levels of ALT were 400 U/l which are extremely high as they should be below 32 U/l.

GTT - (gamma glutamyl transpeptidase) is often elevated in those who use alcohol or other liver toxic substances to excess. An enzyme produced in many tissues as well as the liver. It may be elevated in the serum of patients with bile duct diseases. Her GGT levels were 323 U/l which again were very high as the acceptable parameters are between 5 and 36;

AST - (aspartate aminotransferase) which was previously called SGOT. This is a mitochondrial enzyme that is also present in heart, muscle, kidney and brain therefore it is less specific for liver disease. In many cases of liver inflammation, the ALT and AST activities are elevated roughly in a 1:1 ratio. Her levels were again very elevated at 188 U/l when acceptable parameters should be below 32 U/l.

Bilirubin is the major breakdown product that results from the destruction of old red blood cells (as well as some other sources). It is removed from the blood by the liver, chemically modified by a process call conjugation, secreted into the bile, passed into the intestine and to some extent reabsorbed from the intestine. It is basically the pigment that gives faeces its brown colour. Her levels of Total bilirubin were very high at 4.7 mg/dl when acceptable parameters should be below 1 and her direct bilirubin (see explanation below) was 2.7 when acceptable parameters are closer to zero (0.0 – 0.2).

Elevated levels of bilirubin can mean:

a) Bilirubin concentrations are elevated in the blood either by increased production, decreased uptake by the liver, decreased conjugation (modification to make it water soluble), decreased secretion from the liver or blockage of the bile ducts.

b) In cases of increased production, decreased liver uptake or decreased conjugation, the unconjugated or so-called indirect bilirubin will be primarily elevated.

c) In cases of decreased secretion from the liver or bile duct obstruction, the conjugated or so-called direct bilirubin will be primarily elevated.

AP - (alkaline phosphatase) is elevated in many types of liver disease but also in non-liver related diseases. Alkaline phosphatase is an enzyme, or more precisely a family of related enzymes, that is produced in the bile ducts and sinusoidal membranes of the liver but is also present in many other tissues. An elevation in the level of serum alkaline phosphatase is raised in bile duct blockage from any cause. Her levels were elevated at 137 U/l were acceptable parameters are 35 to 104.

Given that all the blood parameters were pointing to a blockage of the gallbladder duct by calculi, she was strongly advised to remove the gallbladder immediately (cholecystectomy) the same day. She had suffered from gallbladder problems back in 2005 - this was the first time that I saw her and we managed to deal with this using a natural gallbladder flush that cleared all the stones from her gallbladder and her symptoms disappeared. Based on this past experience, she was now adamant to repeat the gallbladder flush again and avoid the cholecystectomy, even though her situation now was a little more pressing than before!

Holistic diagnosis:
Given the time constraints with the current medical and biochemical diagnosis, there were not many tests that were run apart from the Hair Tissue Mineral Analysis. This showed extremely low levels of many minerals including calcium, magnesium, potassium, manganese and cobalt with heavy metals such as mercury, arsenic, cadmium and aluminium appearing in circulation.

Holistic treatments:
As I pointed out to Mrs. K on initial consultation, her situation was a little more critical than previously as there was now an obstruction in the gallbladder ducts that had led to the high hepatic enzymes and the stress on the liver. She was also in acute pain with intense pain in the upper and middle abdomen that would radiate to the right shoulder blade. Pain would be worse after eating and could last a few hours and become very intense at times to the point of feeling nausea. It was an indication of the disruption of bile flow with the bile duct muscles contracting to try to force the bile though the ducts.

There was little time to undergo a series of tests, so I told her that we should begin working on clearing the obstruction using a gallbladder flush that she had done in the past, helping the flow of bile using herbs and supplements, as well as working towards softening the stones with magnesium malate and plenty of apple juice, which contains malic acid. We would monitor the situation closely with the help of the medical doctor who could do further ultrasound scans and blood tests. If all else failed she would go in for surgery, even though she was very determined to avoid it at all costs.

She began a 15-day alkaline detoxification diet with fresh fruit, steamed vegetables, salads, freshly made carrot and green juice and herbal teas on the 8.9.09. She was given a number of nutritional supplements such as a high-potency multivitamin formula, omega 3, 6 and 9 fatty acids to help with the inflammation. Globe artichoke (Cynara scolymus) has been found to increase bile secretion in perfused rat liver and liver cell cultures[33,34] and has been reported in one small double-blind, placebo-controlled trial and several case series to increase choleresis (secretion of bile).[35]

A herbal formula that contained vitamin B1, B6, B12, folic acid (all required for the P-450 Cytochrome detoxication pathways of the liver), N-Acetyl-Cysteine, Trimethylglycine, Scutellaria baicalensis root extract, Milk thistle, Artichoke and Lipoic Acid (a universal fat and water soluble antioxidant to protect the liver against damage). Moreover, she took Aloe Vera juice and vitamin C as calcium ascorbate powder – 2 grams, three times daily to help further in the dissolution of the stones.

Scutellaria baicalensis is a botanical commonly used in Traditional Chinese Medicine. Research has indicated it has many interesting effects on the liver. A number of in vitro and animal studies indicate that Scutellaria baicalensis can improve liver health. A recent cell culture study tested three active flavonoid components of the root of Scutellaria baicalensis on a human liver cancer cell line. The results indicated that the components of Scutellaria baicalensis inhibited the oxidation of protein in the liver and the decrease of cell viability that had occurred in the cancer cells prior to exposure to the botanical compounds. The Scutellaria baicalensis component baicalin had the strongest inhibitory effect. The researchers concluded that all three components of Scutellaria baicalensis could inhibit liver injury in a dose dependent manner.[36]

---

[33] Kraft K. Artichoke leaf extract - Recent findings reflecting effects on lipid metabolism, liver and gastrointestinal tracts. *Phytomedicine* 4(4):369-378, 1997.

[34] Matuschowski P. Testing of Cynara scolymus in the isolated perfused rat liver. 43rd *Ann Congr Soc Med Plant Res* 3-7, 1996.

[35] Kirchhoff R, Beckers CH, Kirchhoff GM, and et al. Increase in choleresis by means of artichoke extract. *Phytomedicine* 1:107-115, 1994.

This same protective effect was seen in a study investigating the use of the Scutellaria baicalensis component baicalin in rats given high doses of acetaminophen. When acetaminophen is given at high doses it is extremely toxic to the liver. In this study, however, when rats were given baicalin a half hour after acetaminophen administration, it significantly prevented many of the toxic effects observed in rats given acetaminophen without baicalin. Furthermore, none of the rats given baicalin with acetaminophen died, whereas 43 percent of the rats given only acetaminophen died. Baicalin also prevented the acetaminophen-related drop in levels of glutathione, a critical antioxidant mentioned below.[37]

N-Acetyl-Cysteine (NAC) is a powerful antioxidant, which increases the production of the critical antioxidant glutathione. Glutathione is the chief chemical used by the liver exerting a variety of protective effects, including detoxification and intracellular defense against oxidative stress. NAC is even used by conventional medicine to treat life threatening acetaminophen poisoning.[38]

Milk Thistle seeds contain a bioflavonoid complex known as silymarin, responsible for the health benefits of the plant. Today, laboratory and clinical tests confirm milk thistle's significant liver-protective effects. A potent antioxidant in its own right, silymarin is particularly remarkable for its beneficial effects on glutathione. Researchers have found that silymarin increases levels of glutathione by up to 35 percent. Silymarin has also been shown to regenerate injured liver cells. In addition, silymarin has the ability to block fibrosis, a process that contributes to the eventual development of cirrhosis.[39]

On 30.9.09, twenty five days after beginning her holistic treatments she had another blood test that showed that her hepatic enzymes had began to reduce; gamma-GT from 324 to 164 (still high); SGOT from 188 to 22 (now in normal range); SGPT from 400 to 60 (still high) – the clinical

---

36 Zhao Y, Li H, Gao Z, Gong Y, Xu H. Effects of flavonoids extracted from Scutellaria baicalensis Georgi on hemin-nitrite-H2O2 induced liver injury. *Eur J Pharmacol*. 24;536(1-2):192-9, Apr 2006.

37 Jang SI, Kim HJ, Hwang KM, Jekal SJ, Pae HO, Choi BM, Yun YG, Kwon TO, Chung HT, Kim YC. Hepatoprotective effect of baicalin, a major flavone from Scutellaria radix, on acetaminophen-induced liver injury in mice. *Immunopharmacol Immunotoxicol*. 25(4):585-94, Nov 2003.

38 Ellenhorn MJ, et al. Ellenhorn's Medical Toxicology: Diagnoses and Treatment of Human Poisoning. 2nd edition. Baltimore, MD. Williams & Wilkins, 1997.

39 Ferenci P, Dragosics B, Dittrich H, et al. Randomized controlled trial of silymarin treatment in patients with cirrhosis of the liver. *J Hepatol*. 9:105-13, 1989.

chemist and medical doctor commented that this was an extremely rapid decline, indicating that the liver was beginning to regain functioning again.

This test was performed 5 days after she had done her first gallbladder flush which removed a number of stones and 25 days into the holistic treatment programme. The blood results were encouraging as all pathological parameters were normalizing and this greatly encouraged her to continue. Besides, she was now feeling a lot better and the pain in the gallbladder region had reduced considerably and she was no longer getting shooting pains into her right shoulder.

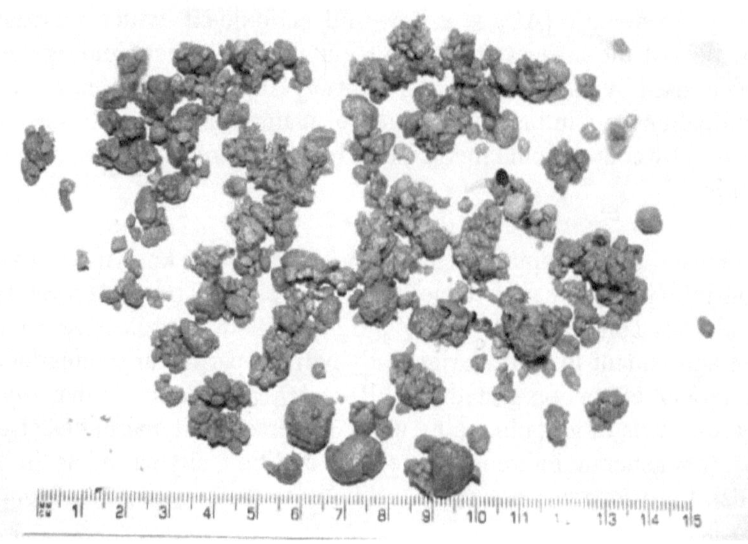

Gallstones flushed the first time

During the gallbladder flush apple juice is taken which is high in malic acid, which is thought to act as a solvent to weaken adhesions between solid globules. Epsom salts (magnesium sulphate) are used because it's believed it relaxes smooth muscle and will relax and dilate the bile duct to enable larger solid particles (like gallstones) to exit the gallbladder. Unrefined olive oil is used to stimulate the gallbladder and bile duct to contract and expel gallstones. The image above shows the number of stones flushed from the gallbladder the first time around.

About 14 days after beginning her holistic treatment protocol she had another ultrasound scan which read: "the gallbladder is not as distended as on the previous examination, but there is now marked thickening of the gallbladder wall with an oedematous ring, indicating inflammation of the gallbladder wall. There is a large cluster of small calculi noted within the gallbladder, which is more clearly evident on today's examination. There are no features of pancreatitis sonographically. The features are suggestive of less obstruction on today's examination, but there is a complication of associated cholecystitis."

The medical doctors again strongly encouraged her to go in for gallbladder surgery, but she was adamant and managed to stall them further. When the gallbladder empties, as had occurred on the first flush, the stones left in the liver ducts will slowly make their way down into the gallbladder again. This can fill with stones AGAIN, and therefore more flushes are required – sometimes as many as 5-6 flushes are required to completely clear all the stones from the liver and gallbladder – therefore the scan showed more stones a couple of weeks after the initial flush. Had the scan been taken only a couple of days after the flush, then the chances are that it would have shown no stones, or very few.

She continued her supplements and towards the end of October 2008 she did another gallbladder flush and removed more smallish stones. Another blood analysis on the 21.10.09 which was a few days after her second gallbladder flush showed a marked decrease in hepatic enzymes back to normal levels: gamma-GT fell from 164 on last count to 36 (now about normal); AST from 188 to 18 (now normal) and ALT from 66 to 23 (now normal). These results had occurred within 6 weeks of beginning her holistic protocol.

Moreover, all the pain had disappeared completely, and she had no further problems after eating. In fact, she had lost considerable weight and her energy levels had greatly increased, her bowel distension was gone and generally she was feeling very well.

Patient's own account:
I have been doing gallbladder flushes for some time, ever since I visited Dr. Georgiou in 2005. However, due to excessive stresses at work and at home, with a hectic lifestyle, I failed to look after myself over the last two to three years, eating anything but an optimum diet, not drinking enough water and generally putting on excess weight. This was not the advice that I received from Dr. Georgiou who mentioned doing a general body detox every 6

months with fruit and vegetables, as well as flushing the gallbladder at least once per year based on my previous history of gallstones.

When I returned to Dr. Georgiou I was in a real state. I had lots of pain in the gut area that kept shooting up to my upper back, I was bloated most of the day and I was afraid to eat as the pain would get worse. I was also feeling tired and run down, so I went to see a medical doctor first to see whether it was what I suspected, gallstones again. Indeed, the ultrasound scan confirmed this, as did the blood tests where all my liver enzymes were sky high! When the doctor had completed his examination, he was determined to get me into surgery the same day and actually called the surgeon there and then to book me an appointment that afternoon.

Even though I was worried as I knew that this was serious, I always had faith in natural medicine as I and my family had relied on it for many years and I really did not want my gallbladder whipped out. Over the years I have developed a sort of "allergy" towards medical doctors due to many of the mistakes and consequences that I have seen in other friends and family members.

I therefore called Dr. Georgiou who is normally very busy and puts you on a waiting list, but as soon as he heard my voice he recognized me and luckily he had a cancellation the same day. I did not hesitate and got my husband to drive me to Larnaca where we met. He looked at the results with a worried frown and said after a few minutes, well it looks like you are really close to surgery – why are you here? How can I help?

I told him quite categorically that I had no intention of being put under the knife and that I wanted to do another gallbladder flush under his supervision. He continued to tell me that my liver was under considerable stress as the liver enzymes had shot up, possibly because of an obstruction of the gallbladder ducts. However, he said that if we moved quickly and monitored the situation with the help of the medical doctor, we would see. He said that he had a similar case and they had succeeded, but each case has its own individual qualities. He said that the reassuring thing was that he knew me from previous consultations and that I was a good and well-behaved patient.

He immediately put me on an alkaline detoxification diet with supplements to help reduce my liver enzymes, as well as others to soften the gallbladder stones and asked to see me in a weeks' time. By that time, I began to feel better, so we decided to implement the first gallbladder cleanse which went well with no pain or complications. A few days later the blood tests had confirmed that my liver was improving by leaps and bounds and this was really encouraging. Dr. Georgiou advised that I continue the supplements and plan for another gallbladder flush soon.

By the time I completed the second flush I was a new woman – all the pains had gone, as well as the bloating – I was eating normally now but within a more optimal diet (I got my knuckles wrapped by Dr. Georgiou on this), my energy and stamina had much increased and so had my overall moods which were much happier. My blood tests also showed that my liver enzymes were normal, which relieved me considerably as this was very worrying. Dr. Georgiou was also again smiling!

I was elated and very happy to have saved myself the ordeal and expense of gallbladder surgery. I am also grateful to Dr. Georgiou for his faith in natural medicine and the results that it can bring to many patients like me. He really is a most caring and committed practitioner that finds amazing ways of getting people well, even with critical cases like mine.

Dr. Georgiou's final comments on Mrs. K:
This was a most interesting case where natural medicine showed its power by healing the liver and gallbladder in a very short period of time. Even though I have personally supervised hundreds of gallbladder flushes, this one was a little "on the edge" due to the high liver enzymes and the possible blockage. However, with a positive attitude, a healthy optimism and a systematic approach, having faith in the power of natural healing remedies, as well as the innate healing forces of the body, it is amazing how healing miracles are performed.

It is important to state here that patients facing similar crises should not simply take their treatments into their own hands without the supervision of an experienced holistic practitioner, who will work with other medical specialists to carefully monitor the patient every step of the way.

Disclaimer

The information contained within this book is offered in order for you to make educated health decisions so that you can optimize your health. If there are serious health conditions, then you should always consult your primary care physician before beginning any other treatment regime.

The health information in this book is not advice and should not be treated as such – it is provided without any representations or warranties, express or implied. We do not warrant or represent that the medical information in this book is true, accurate, complete, current or non-misleading.

You must not rely on the information in this book as an alternative to medical advice from your doctor or other professional healthcare provider. If you have any specific questions about any medical matter, you should consult your doctor or other professional healthcare provider. If you think you may be suffering from any medical condition, you should seek immediate medical attention. You should never delay seeking medical advice, disregard medical advice or discontinue medical treatment because of information in this book.

While every attempt has been made to provide information that is both accurate and cutting-edge, the author and publisher cannot be held responsible for any decision that the reader may take while reading the guide, nor can a guarantee be provided that this guide and the remedies that it recommends will help everyone.

CONSULTATIONS & FURTHER EDUCATION

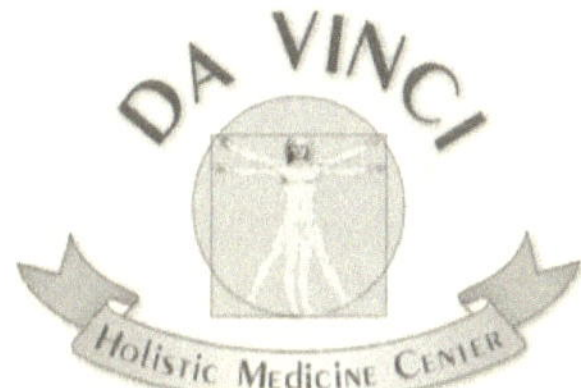

Clinical Consultations
To book appointments to see Dr Georgiou at the Da Vinci Holistic Health Center in Larnaca, Cyprus simply call the Center or email.

Tel: +357 24 – 82 33 22
Email: admin@naturaltherapycenter.com
Web: www.naturaltherapycenter.com

Da Vinci Institute of Holistic Medicine

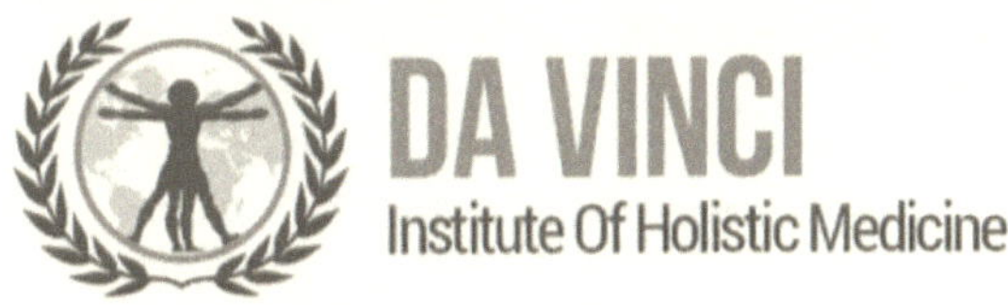

Anyone interested in completing studies in Holistic Medicine can apply directly to the Da Vinci Institute.
Tel: +357 24 – 82 33 22

Email: admin@collegenaturalmedicine.com
Web: www.collegenaturalmedicine.com

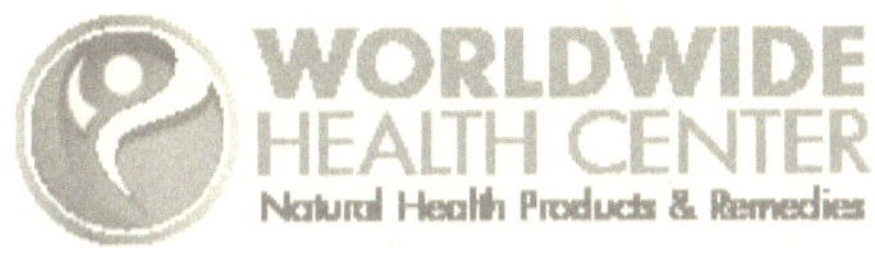

Worldwide Health Center
Most of the supplements mentioned in this book can be obtained from this website.
Tel: +357 24 82 33 22

Email: admin@worldwidehealthcenter.net
Web: www.worldwidehealthcenter.net

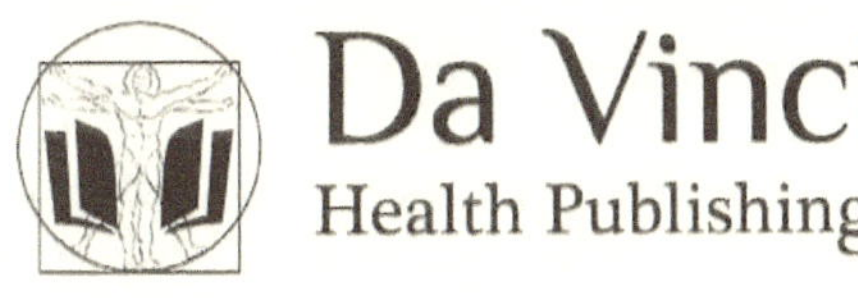

Da Vinci Health Publishing
Health practitioners that want to publish their books, but do not want to lose their copyright, while gaining most of the
royalties, can apply to Da Vinci Health Publishing – the ethical publishers!
Tel: + 357 24 82 33 22
Email: admin@davincipublishers.com

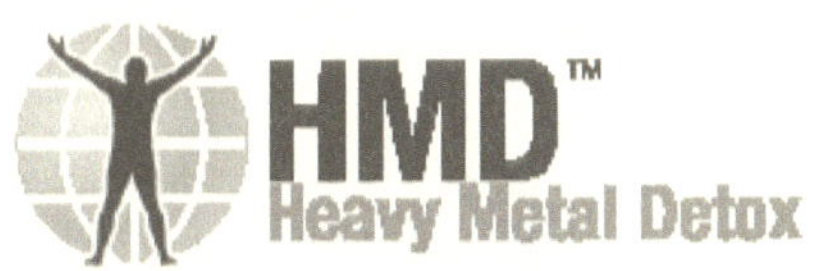

Detox Heavy Metals
Products related to the natural detox of toxic metals can be purchased here - sent globally.
Tel: + 357 24 82 33 22

Email: admin@detoxmetals.com
Web: www.detoxmetals.com

ABOUT THE AUTHOR

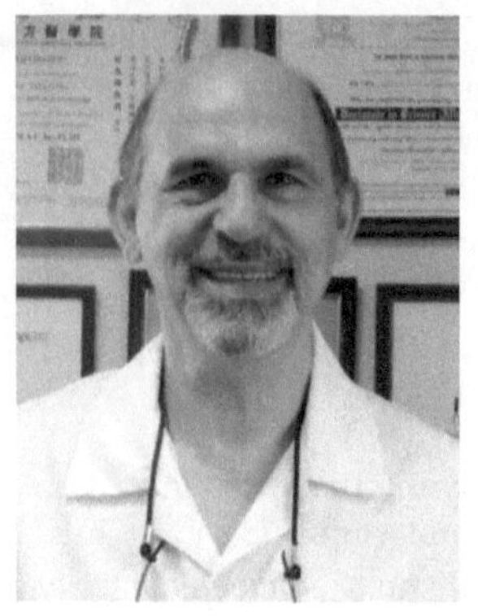

Dr. George John Georgiou, 62 years old, has 11 degrees and Diplomas spanning 25 years in various topics ranging from Biology, Psychology and Natural Medicine. Specifically:

1. Bachelor of Science (B.Sc) honours degree in Biology/Psychology from Oxford Brook's University, Oxford, England
2. Master's of Science degree (M.Sc) in Clinical Psychology from the University of Surrey, Guildford, England
3. Doctor of Philosophy degree (Ph.D). in Clinical Sexology from The Institute for Advanced Study of Human Sexuality, San Francisco, USA.
4. Doctor of Science (D.Sc (AM)) degree in Alternative Medicine from the International Open University of Alternative Medicine
5. Clinical Nutrition (Dip.ION - Distinction) from the Institute of Optimum Nutrition (ION), London, England
6. Diploma in Electronic Impulse Therapy (Dip.E.I.Th) from the Euro College of Complementary Medicine, UK
7. Diploma in Naturopathic Iridology from the Holistic Health College, UK and Diploma in Iridology from the Society of Iridologists, UK
8. Diploma as a Master Herbalist (MH) from the Holistic Health College, UK
9. Diploma in Homeopathic Medicine (DIHom) from the British Institute of Homeopathy, UK
10. Diploma in Su Jok Acupuncture from Onnuri College, Almaty, Kazakhstan
11. Doctor of Naturopathic Medicine (Pastoral) – N.D. (P) from the Sacred Medical Order of the Knights of Hope, US – Licence number: L1016988.

He is the Director Founder of the Da Vinci Holistic Health Centre in Larnaca, Cyprus – see www.naturaltherapycenter.com This is a multimodality centre specializing in treating chronic diseases of all kinds. This model of healthcare using a holistic approach has been illustrated in his 23 books that he has written to date.

Research is also one of his passions and he is considered an expert in natural heavy metals detoxification, having been awarded a Doctor of Science in this topic. He has spent over three years formulating and testing using double-blind, placebo-controlled trials with over 350 people a natural toxic metal chelator called HMD™

(Heavy Metal Detox). He is presently the worldwide patent-pending holder on this product which is sold worldwide at www.detoxmetals.com

There are many papers that Dr Georgiou has published in peer-reviewed journals that are available on his websites at www.naturaltherapycenter.com and www.detoxmetals.com

Dr Georgiou has also been Knighted as a Knight Hospitaller by the Sovereign Medical Order of the Knights Hospitaller (www.smokh.org), one of the oldest Christian charitable organizations in the world with over 200 medical knights all practicing holistic medicine using natural medicine formulated by the monks of old practicing monastic medicine. They have built 5 hospitals and clinics worldwide all running on charitable donations to help the poor. As the Diplomatic Cultural Attache for Cyprus he is presently in the process of setting up such a charitable clinic in Larnaca, Cyprus where he lives and works.

His research interests have made him the Principle Investigator for the World Health Organization (WHO) in studies on AIDS and Drug Use, as well as other research involving alcoholism, drug abuse and sexual dysfunctions. He has lectured to Masters students in Psychology at an external campus for Indiana University, USA, and has been a prolific writer of health articles for the general public, having written literally thousands in both English and Greek languages.

Regarding his career in Clinical Sexology, he was the first professional sexologist to ever work in Cyprus, making history in this respect. This was back in 1983 when sexology was unheard of in this sexually repressed country.

His doctoral dissertation in Clinical Sexology was entitled *The Sexual Attitudes of Greek Orthodox Priests* – a unique study never before studied in the Orthodox religion. There was considerable antagonism from certain spheres of the Orthodox Greek church regarding the results of the study.

In 1990 he had his own live radio programme on Saturday lunchtime entitled *Human Sexuality*. This was far ahead of its time and in a two-year period Dr Georgiou managed to cover 96 topics of human sexuality with the audience asking questions reflecting the ignorance, taboos and prejudices of the time. This was the first such programme in the history of Cyprus.

In 1999 he published the first book ever written in the Greek language on the treatment of Premature Ejaculation, published in Greece. He is also the Editor for the chapter on Cyprus in the International Encyclopedia of Sexuality, Volume 4.

As Dr Georgiou has two doctorates, one in Clinical Sexology and one in Alternative Medicine, he has formulated protocols for the treatment of sexual dysfunctions that involve the integration of both these disciplines. He has coined this *Naturopathic Sexology* which is a unique term pertinent to himself – if you Google this term it will bring you back to his websites.

He is presently the Director Founder of the Da Vinci Holistic Health Center in Larnaca, Cyprus, as well as the Academic Director of the Da Vinci College of Holistic Medicine, a distance-learning educational institution, and the Director/founder of the Da Vinci BioSciences Research Center.

He is a Member of the following Associations/Institutes:

- The Society of Biology, UK (MSBiol.)
- Chartered Biologist, UK (C. Biol)
- Member of the Royal Microscopy Society, UK
- The General Council and Register of Naturopaths, UK (GCRN)
- Full Member, The British Naturopathic Association, UK
- Member of Oncology Group, British Naturopathic Association
- The Register of Naturopathic Iridologists, UK (M.R.N.I.)
- The British Association of Nutritional Therapists, UK (BANT)
- The Association of Master Herbalists, UK. (AMH)
- Fellow of the British Institute of Homeopathy, UK (FBIH)
- The American College of Clinical Thermology, USA
- The International Su Jok Therapy Association, Russia
- The British Holistic Medical Association, UK (BHMA)
- Member of the Institute of Complementary Medicine, UK (ICM)
- National Iridology Research Association, USA (NIRA)
- Associate Fellow of the British Psychological Society, UK (AFBPsS)
- Chartered Psychologist, UK, BPS (C.Psychol)
- Member, Health Professions Council, UK – registered as Clinical Psychologist (PYL15128)
- Member of Cyprus Psychologists' Association, Cyprus.
- Diplomate of the American Board of Sexology, USA (ABS)
- Registered Sex Therapist with ABS, USA
- Member, The American College of Sexologists, USA (ACS)
- Fellow of the American Academy of Clinical Sexologists, USA (FAACS)
- Member, World Association for Sexology (WAS), USA
- Member of the Cyprus Association of Alternative Therapists (N.D.).

Dr. Georgiou is married to Maria, a Psychotherapist/Lecturer and has 4 children aged between 18 and 31 years. His hobbies and interests include flying a private plane, classic antique motorbike and car restoration, antique furniture restoration, playing the bouzouki, horology, web master, travelling, writing, running his private lab specialising in energy medicine, molecular biology and microbiology, bee keeping and running an organic farm.

More Books written by Dr Georgiou:

1. Surviving a Nuclear War: Save Your Family and Loved Ones
2. Candida Cure: Healing Naturally in 90-Days – 5,000 Successful Cases!
3. Diabetes: Natural Treatments that Really Work – Latest Research!
4. Crohn's Disease: Heal Naturally Without Medication
5. Reflux Disease: Natural Healing for GERD in 90 Days
6. Lupus: Let Nature Heal – Find Out How
7. Haemorrhoids: The Natural Cure
8. Cholesterol: Heal Naturally Without Medication – Many Secrets Revealed!
9. Diverticulosis: Natural Healing That Works
10. Why Am I Sick? Eliminate the Causes and Be Well Forever!